The Chronicles of Nausea

A Diary of Hyperemesis Gravidarum

D1466610

Ashli Foshee McCall

Table of Contents

To every mother who has suffered the isolation, alienation, and torture that is hyperemesis gravidarum.

Preface

When I started this book it wasn't a book at all. It was actually a blog that I'd set up in 2003 for the purpose of giving the public an intimate glimpse of what it means to live with severe hyperemesis gravidarum (HG). I have come to accept that the general population regards HG as "a little puking." But those of us who have had this illness know better. While the prevailing attitude regarding HG stems from the good news that pregnancy is normal for most people, unrealistic perceptions can contribute not only to the poor treatment of sufferers but also to the isolation we feel when the horror of our everyday experience is underestimated.

Hopefully, this diary will promote HG awareness and education, validate the experience, and reassure sufferers. I wrote *Beyond Morning Sickness* and *Mama Has Hyperemesis Gravidarum* for the same reasons. I had planned to publish another book, regarding Biblical reflections on HG, but I don't know that I will be able to meet that goal.

In 2009 I was diagnosed with pancreatic neuroendocrine cancer (pNET), the cancer that took the life of Apple's Steve Jobs. Approximately three in 1,000,000 people receive this diagnosis annually.[1] Whether there is some medical reason that I am

---

1 Yao JC An update on pancreatic neuroendocrine tumors
Retrieved September 9, 2012 from
http://www.oncologystat.com

prone to rare illnesses is uncertain. What I am sure of is the fact that my cancer diagnosis reinforces my view that nothing has affected me as physically, emotionally, and spiritually as HG. I am dealing with a disease that may become terminal, but it is only a troubling footnote to my existence, not my life's cause. It never will be, because new cases of HG are diagnosed each day in this country, and I know what that means.

While it is true that friends and family have wondered aloud whether my pregnancies, diet or even mysterious environmental exposures caused my cancer, no one has ever suggested that my tumor was perhaps a physical manifestation of mental illness, that I employ a positive attitude in order to somehow "think" it away, or that I try harder not to have it. The diagnosis did not make anyone question my integrity. The tumor was there; it was something the doctors could see, and therefore it was real. Consequently, no one ever inferred that I had cancer because somewhere in the deep recesses of my mind I didn't really want to be alive. I had a disease that needed treatment. That is all. Being a cancer patient is a very different experience.

The personal dismissal that many HG patients encounter is genuine and unfair. Battling cancer only confirms this; it has wiped away any private doubt that HG patients, in particular, are victimized by those who hold mistaken ideas. Perhaps knowledge will someday afford relief. I have done my best to contribute to that effort.

We must fight the good fight together, never forgetting the women who come after us, never letting them suffer alone. They must see our success and know without a doubt that it can be their own.

Ashli Foshee McCall
December 27, 2012

September

Monday, September 22, 2003

I have had hyperemesis gravidarum three times.

I am now pregnant for the fourth time and expect to get HG, although I am willing to suspend certainty. However, I'm five weeks and feel it coming on.

They say there are four things you're supposed to do when you're seeking God's will with a particular issue: pray, read the Bible, consult other trusted Christians, and examine the opportunities set before you. We did all this, endeavored, and are pregnant. I hope we did what we were supposed to do. So there's the explanation for those of you who know me and are going, "What in the heck were you thinking?!"

I was thinking that I could do all things, live or die or suffer like a dog, with Christ. I was thinking that if it was OK with Him, I'd maybe go for it. We'd like for our son not to be a "lonely only." And I want another baby butt to diaper. Children=joy. More children=more joy. This is me attempting to justify what normal women are never asked to justify. But I *am* a normal woman. It's my *body* that won't cooperate.

And so it begins.

I took three pregnancy tests that I bought online. One: negative. Two: negative. Three: negative. Why all these pregnancy tests? Because I was feeling kinda barfy before I even missed a period. Negative, negative, negative. I went to a doctor's appointment. They wanted to do X-rays. I said, "I can't, I'm pregnant."

What? I took three negative pregnancy tests. Why would I say that? I clarified, "I mean I might be." I was beginning to think I needed a shrink, because it seemed I couldn't accept the results of three pregnancy tests. But still, no X-rays, thank you.

Three days after the missed period I was feeling even more barfy, and where was the period? Forget the cheap online pregnancy tests. I went to the store and shelled out the big bucks for a pee-on stick.

At home the positive sign popped up in seconds. I retested with a pregnancy strip I bought online. It said negative. Sheesh. I wrote the company. X-rays aren't so bad, but what if I'd seen a dermatologist during that period of time and started taking tetracycline or something? Be careful about buying cheap tests online. Pay the big bucks for the ones at the drugstore.

I've been eating like a cow, indulging in expensive restaurants several times a week. I know what is coming. I'm open to complete and total healing, but I know the illness could be a necessary part of my life journey, so I'm open to that too. Whatever happens, happens. But I'm eating my head off, because if HG returns I know there will be a day when I'd pay a thousand dollars just to be able to eat a sandwich.

I'm going to try to keep a diary. I have a laptop in the bedroom. The hospital bed and overbed table are coming just in case. Still, some days I know there will be no way I will have the strength to get online. I'll try, because it's important that people know what HG is like for the mother who suffers every single moment of every single day.

Today I woke up barfy. It's the barfiest I've been in this pregnancy. I'd say I was at a three on a scale of 1-10. That may not sound like much, but I am pretty conservative in my ratings, and I can go from three to barf in about two seconds. I haven't barfed yet. I'm pretending I might not. I am doing my best to be open to the proposals of some psychological researchers who say HG in subsequent pregnancies could be a learned response. It's suspect, but I'm going give the theory a chance: every time I feel barfy I tell myself I'm not one of Pavlov's dogs.

As I say, I can still eat, although I feel that slipping away. Foods don't sound immediately good. Eatables are starting to give me the creeps. Still, if I ingest something I feel better for about 10 minutes or so. This must be what it's like to be a normal pregnant woman. I know a number of women who were not at all ill during their many pregnancies, but that sort of thing actually exists at the other end of the spectrum of "abnormal."

I am monitoring my fluids closely. I know how important this is for HG moms. Keeping it together today means staving it off a little while longer before it becomes fully out of control.

I am planning to take ondansetron (Zofran) for the first time. I think this will be interesting, as I've had a tendency to sort of secretly discount it due to the studies I've read on HG and serotonin. Serotonin doesn't appear to be implicated, and ondansetron is a serotonin receptor antagonist. Explain *that*. However, I cannot deny the many positive Zofran experiences that other sufferers report.

In addition to HG, I have an incompetent cervix (IC), so cerclage will be performed. HG doesn't go well with an IC. Nothing that puts pressure on the cervix is good especially as the pregnancy progresses. I'm also considering corticosteroids for the HG at around 15 weeks if I haven't miscarried. Even with the cerclage I will remain on strict bed rest and will have to walk up and down the hall three times a day to try to avoid potentially fatal blood clots.

Fun.

I have never "done" HG while having to take care of another child. I will hopefully be able to use this diary to explore the experience. I imagine HG is a *lot* harder with other children. In fact, I've been contacted on several occasions by women who terminated the second child because they felt they could not take care of the first. It is especially difficult for single mothers.

Any and all prayers are welcome for *all* women with HG, and my name is Ashli for your prayer chains and lists at church.

I will keep you posted as I am able.

Wednesday, September 24, 2003

Yesterday I had a period of time that was roughly a six on my 1-10 nausea scale. No sir, I didn't like it. Right now I seem to be able to eat and stave off the barfiness just like the pregnancy books say. Evidently, this is how it works for normal women. It is still an all-day battle. This time I am finding that sleep nullifies the effects of nausea. Sometimes my sleeping son will nudge me until I'm half awake, and for a brief moment of awareness I think, "Hmmm, I'm not nauseous at all." But when I awake fully the nausea starts in. This would support the neurological theories that HG is based on a malfunction of the "vomiting center" in the brain. Sedate the brain and that sort of shuts it off. This is part of the reason why women with HG are given sedatives, such as Phenergan and Thorazine, as antiemetics (puke-stoppers). The only problem with the theory is that the drug therapies aren't very effective. In fact, the drugs can actually make it worse. Theories are fun—when you're not sick.

Last night I drank a milkshake. First, praise God, I could drink a milkshake! It was really freakily effective in quelling the nausea. It lasted for a good 15 minutes before I was climbing back up to a level four or so. Still no puking! By week six it's going to be "on." Unless God shuts it off. ("Hey, God! Please shut the puke switch off! Pretty please, with Zofran on top!") I just had another milkshake to try to quell the nausea as I type this. It's not working like it did last night.

Eating is becoming troublesome. Foods that I know are delicious don't taste delicious, and I'm starting to have to sort of choke it all down. It is hard not to be afraid. It is hard to live for today and not be daunted by the months that stretch out ahead. If it were just like it is today there would be no problem. But HG is not here yet. Today the battle is cake, but it can get so very much worse.

I cried yesterday wondering what I had gotten myself into. I knew there would be days when I would feel incredibly stupid for inviting all of this into our lives again. Yesterday I was already having those thoughts, and this nausea I'm dealing with is *nothing* compared to HG, so it's distressing. What I'm going through now would probably be very significant to a normal woman, but I have something to compare it to. Something that was so bad that it compelled me to pay a terrible price in order to escape it.

I can feel HG coming. It's like a big dog barking in the distance. But God is bigger. Sometimes it is hard to remember in deep suffering, but I must never forget.

Thursday, September 25, 2003

Whoa, Nelly! How much longer until the puking begins? I thought for sure I'd be gone by yesterday, but I held it together and even managed to eat dinner. I waded through the day on peanut butter and jelly sandwiches and three milkshakes. By dinner I wanted Chinese. Stinky, smelly, greasy Chinese. Eat it while you can. I wasn't sure about this meal choice, but it went down and stayed down, and I felt like a new person. It was hard to keep from crying all through dinner, because I was so utterly grateful. I'm teary-eyed just remembering it.

This morning I woke up throbbing with nausea. Quick, get something in me. Make it stop. I choked down a quarter of a peanut butter and jelly sammy. I'm already sick of that, but it's all I can stand right now. Smells are bothering me. Don't cook it whatever it is. Bread toasting in the oven? Don't make me hurl.

I've been amazed that eating quells anything. I don't remember it ever doing so before. It could have been so, in previous pregnancies, in the early weeks leading up to HG, but perhaps I've forgotten. Or perhaps it's different this time. It feels like things are progressing.

I just ate something an hour ago, and it didn't do much of anything to help. I had a drink with it, and you're not supposed to do that. You're supposed to wait an hour after solids. I was thirsty. I want to drink while I still have the pleasure of experiencing thirst, before the notion of drinking turns into an unthinkable horror. In former pregnancies I got so dehydrated that my lips cracked and bled, but just the suggestion of consuming fluid sent me to the toilet puking.

Soon, by week six I think, I'll begin unraveling. Already the hopelessness is seeping in and the attitude of "I don't want to do this! What an insane, idiotic idea this was!" I *can't* be feeling this defeated so early in the game; my symptoms are trivial compared to what they could become!

If I think of the days ahead, the weeks ahead, 16 more of them (because I usually resolve by 20 weeks), and take them all in one lump sum, I realize I have about 112 days left. That's 2,688 more hours of existing this way and worse. I can feel an acid scream rising in my throat. I can feel the fear. The desperation sets in. But somehow, God is here.

I am not alone.

Saturday, September 27, 2003

The nausea cranked up to about a seven or eight on the scale and just hung there. Yesterday I pseudo-puked for the first time. I.e., I got out of bed and retched over the toilet but nothing came out. Not so lucky this morning.

I woke up and thought I could choke down an Ensure to perhaps stave off the bad nausea and puking. I got it down alright—only to puke it up 15 minutes later. After that lovely episode I took a shower thinking it would clean me up and relax me. Hello! What was I thinking? Thermal changes relaxing? I puked up the rest of the Ensure in the shower. The bottom of the stall filled with chocolate puke, and that just made me puke even more.

I got in the bed and cried.

I'm already hoping I miscarry. What hyperemetic doesn't? I see where all this is going. I see the year-long days stretching out before me like a round-the-world journey. I try to live moment by moment, but it is so hard not to get daunted by what is ahead: fear coupled with 24/7 nausea and vomiting. I don't *want* to go down this road. I don't feel as committed as before. And yet, there's nothing in the world I can do about it. Nothing I *will* do about it, although the unthinkable thought has crossed my mind in nauseating daydreams.

I took some Zofran for the first time about three hours ago. I took it because my doctor wouldn't prescribe an anti-nausea wristband that emits small electric shocks at set intervals. His reason: he doesn't know enough about it. So here I am online gleaning info to justify my request for non-pharmaceutical treatment. But I'm already on Zofran at less than six weeks. Great.

After I took the Zofran I fell asleep. I woke up an hour later with searing anxiety. It reminded me of Reglan. Does Zofran cause extrapyramidal effects? I'll have to read through my research. Do I need Benadryl? Ah, more drugs. Great.

My husband was taking our tot to Grandma's when I woke up. I tried to hold it together, but I just got overwhelmed, unable to see one more day of this suffering. This, along with the bizarre anxiety, had me walking up and down the hall weeping.

The awful part: this is nothing. Nothing at all what it could be.

And yet it's the worst.

It is here, and it's happening to me.

Sunday, September 28, 2003

I am no longer eating. Yesterday I was able to take in five to six cups of fluid.

I don't see how I'm going to do this. It feels unbearable. I have seriously started hoping for a miscarriage so this can be over. I just want my life back. I just want to be my son's mommy again.

I hate abortion. Anyone who knows me knows how seriously I loathe it. But I have thought about it. God help me I have. I have even gone so far as to look up abortion mills in the Yellow Pages. Horrible. Shocking.

This is illness and desperation. *Desperate* desperation. It has only been three days of puking this time. On top of the years of puking I've done it just seems like too much. This was a very bad idea.

It is easy to feel that God is near, it is easy to be faithful when you are happy and well or are going through certain trials that don't just take everything from you. Now I'm thumbing through abortion listings. Unfathomable.

Will I rob another child of life? Will I deny that I know Christ again? How can I help it? What ever shall I do here, now, in this dreadful situation?

October

Wednesday, October 01, 2003

I have been in the hospital. I just got back yesterday. I tried to get online and write an entry but I was puking as I was typing, so I had to go. I ended up vomiting over 40 times throughout the day. That is to say, I threw up every eight minutes from the moment I woke up in the morning to the moment I went to sleep last night. I stopped counting after the 40th episode. It pains me to admit this, but I was *ready* to abort. Can you believe it? **ME.** This illness is unbelievable. I know I must fight. Sometimes I'm too weak and others have to save me (and my baby) from myself. When I start talking "smack" my husband has learned to take a stand, talk me out of it, **just say no.** He learned this the hard way.

I am only six weeks. I'm on home IVs, and my first vein has already blown. I haven't eaten any type of solid food in five days and have not had even four glasses of fluid to drink in four days. I have never been this sick this soon.

I can't sleep. I have had 11 hours of sleep in the last 72 hours. Nights are the worst. I am *begging* to end it at night. I am begging, unbelievably, to *kill* my very much wanted child. It is not something I want to do. Even in my desperation I know it violates my ethics. But sometimes that knowledge isn't enough. That doesn't make it right. The bottom line is: *I MUST NOT DO IT.*

Please, please pray for me; I'm in the "belly of the whale."

Monday, October 06, 2003

I'm seven weeks. Hospitals, ER visits, insanity. Bleeding last night. Thought maybe miscarriage, but the bleeding stopped, and I'm still puking right along. I haven't eaten food in 11 days. Still not drinking. Still on home IVs. Losing weight (8 pounds so far). If I can't eat soon, if I lose 14 more pounds, I will have to go on a peripherally inserted central catheter (PICC line). This will be fed into a vein in my elbow, threaded up this vein, around my shoulder and down into my chest where it will rest in the part of the heart called the superior vena cava. This will drip feeding solution into my bloodstream and keep me and the baby from starving to death. It can cause serious problems, so I'm not looking forward to it, but I have to try to survive.

Ptyalism is here for the first time: I can't swallow my own spit or I vomit. I have to spit in a cup all day long. Ah, the joys of lying in a bed, vomiting while peeing and pooping on myself (I puke that hard) all while collecting a big cup of smelly viscid spit! All pregnant women envy me.

Can't write more now. Feeling too bad.

Monday, October 13, 2003

On Friday we went to the doctor. The spotting returned, and I showed him the blood so he could get an idea of the amount. He said he considered it to be an impending miscarriage and could perform a D&C if I wanted. I rationalized this notion as acceptable, and yet something stopped me: I know myself, and I believed that if we carried this out I would always feel that I hadn't known for sure that I was miscarrying. And if I wasn't in the middle of a miscarriage, then a D&C was actually an abortion. When it came down to it, I couldn't accept that possibility. I *really* wanted this pregnancy to be over, so it was painful for me to have to tell the doctor that I couldn't do the D&C unless I was certain that I was actively miscarrying. He told me we could be sure by counting the hCG over a period of days. Since it was Friday, we opted to have the second part of the testing done at the emergency room over the weekend in order to get the results faster. I wanted out of this pregnancy as soon as humanly possible, *if* possible.

In the waiting room I lay my head in my husband's lap. I was so relieved to think this could be over soon. A police officer came into the E.R. needing fluids after suffering from a bad virus. Always prepared, our car was packed with bags of IV fluids, and we joked that he could have all he wanted. He and his wife asked why we were in the E.R., and when we told them, they were sad and sorry for us. I explained that as much as we wanted the baby the related health issues were intolerable and so it was actually a relief. They expressed condolences anyway. As we talked, a couple entered the E.R. from inside the hospital. The wife was in a medical gown, her husband at her side. She was walking. Walking is said to bring on or speed up labor, and she was obviously nine months pregnant. I watched in silence. They were adorable and so obviously happy. I was surprised by the evaporation of my relief and the speed with which I found my sadness. I looked at my husband and whispered an apology. Watching that happy couple waddle across the finish line made us feel the somber reality of our situation. It was a little difficult to regain the more practical feeling of relief.

The medical staff called my name, and after a simple blood draw we were on our way home. If the numbers went down instead of up it meant I was in the process of miscarrying. If the numbers doubled it meant the pregnancy was progressing. The doctor called us later with the results: My hCG is skyrocketing, and our baby is not in the process of being miscarried. We don't know what the bleeding means, but it seems to have stopped again. I realize my hell is only beginning, and I mourn for the physical relief I can't have, but I am very grateful that I didn't do the D&C, because now I know for sure what that really would have been.

Thursday, October 30, 2003

A while back I actually had to call an EMT buddy of mine and ask him to come over to start an IV line for me when my home health care nurse couldn't do it. If not for my buddy I would have gone a whole night and part of a day without fluids, which would have meant even more nausea and vomiting. That's not something I want to think about.

But all that's over now. I finally got a PICC line, which means no more blown veins, traumatic multi-sticks to start a new IV or complete failures to do so from nervous home health care nurses. I also got a Zofran pump, so I no longer have to struggle with the foul dissolvable pill, and the effect of the drug can remain more constant. The Zofran pump was a snap. The PICC line wasn't easy.

I was allergic to the material in the first line and had horrible phlebitis, which required line removal. Four days later the second line was placed in the other arm and involved several failed attempts, because I was so dehydrated. No one on a PICC should be dehydrated. But I was. Why? Because my HMO caseworker refused to approve a mechanical pump to go with my first PICC, and I was sent home on a gravity drip. The literature from the hospital's IV therapy (IVT) team states that pumps are not optional. These PICC lines are so long that they can't be gravity fed; the fluids slow down. The techs called my HMO caseworker and explained to her that a mechanical pump was necessary, period. She would not relent. My husband threatened to call an attorney. She approved the pump. It would come to me sometime after I got home, and a home health care nurse would hook it up.

The home health care nurse drove for half an hour to connect my computerized ambulatory drug delivery (CADD) pump.

Upon arrival she remarked that she'd never been taught how to use one, didn't know how it worked, didn't feel comfortable handling it, but would try if I really wanted her to. I sent her away immediately. Someone came out later who actually knew what a mechanical pump was and how to work it. Voila, PICC number two. Which I was also allergic to and which had to be pulled a few days later.

The third PICC came along without much ado. I am told it is an older type of line made of a different material. I must not be allergic to it; it's holding nicely. Still, to have had three PICCs in 10 days is kinda crazy, but I got through it all. The deed is done. The fluids are finally flowin'.

The dressing needs to be changed regularly. You guessed it—home health care nurses do it. These changes are supposed to be as sterile as possible due to the risk of infection in a line that enters the body and ends very near the heart. Such an infection can be serious. When they change the dressing you can't even keep your head straight; you are supposed to turn your face so you are not breathing over your exposed site. I learned that taking my eyes off the procedure was risky when one of the nurses proceeded to change my site with her bare hands. After her visit I got paranoid and called the company that employs her to ask them what the proper procedure was. They told me that nurses definitely must wear gloves. I reported that mine had not and really began to worry. Later the company called me saying they had spoken to the nurse who totally denied changing my site barehanded. I was livid and asked them why, in my debilitated state, I would use what little energy I had to call and stir up trouble if it was baseless. They informed me that it was merely a case of my word against hers. But I know what I saw. She never put on gloves. She took off the plastic dressing and touched the skin around my site with bare fingers. The nurse put me at risk, and her company was not willing to believe the patient or re-educate the employee. I fired them on the spot. Matria (home health company that specializes in HG care) helped me to find another local company that would provide this service, and I am looking forward to working with a nurse who really knows her craft, so that I can finally relax and follow proper procedure myself. When you are an HG patient it seems little comes without a fight.

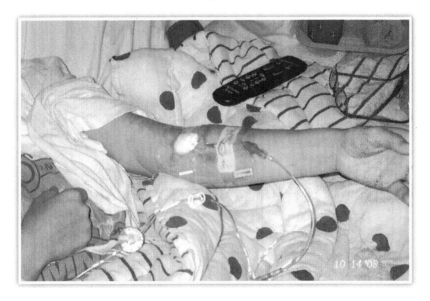

PICC 1: Near my closed hand you can see the flow dial, which indicates a gravity drip—a big no-no for a PICC line. You can also see the drink tray holding my ptyalism cup. YUCK!

PICC

(Peripherally Inserted Central Venous Catheter inserted by Radiology: Non Groshong Catheters)

- A physician's order is needed for placement.
- A STAT portable chest xray is needed to verify tip placement before PICC can be used.
- The PICC is a central line even though it is inserted in the anticubital fossa. You should use these lines the same way you would for a conventional central line.
- These lines must be flushed with three cc's of 10u/cc heparin.
- Apply positive turbulent flush with these lines using nothing smaller than a 10-cc syringe.
- Do not use force to flush these lines.
- These lines cannot be used for radiological procedures using a high-pressure infusor.
- All fluids and medication must be administered through a mechanical pump device.
- It is **not recommended** that blood be drawn through these lines. If no other site is available, call IVT for assistance.
- Do not use alcohol or acetone around the bio-occlusive dressing or catheter.
- IVT will change dressings on PICC lines or those personnel who have been properly trained to do so.
- Monitor the patient for any changes in respiration's or complaints of palpation's/ chest pain.
- Observe and report to IVT any redness, swelling or complaint of discomfort in arm with PICC line.
- If a pump beeps occlusion, flush catheter immediately. If unable to resolve problem or flush, call IVT.

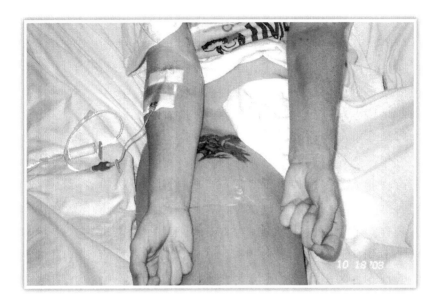

PICC 2: The cluster of failed insertion attempts appears as a dot above my elbow, near the top of the yellow part of my shirt. The Zofran pump catheter is in my tattooed thigh. Unfortunately, I was sitting on the actual pump, and it's under my big, fat butt in the picture. The pump looks like a small, soft eyeglasses case.

November

Wednesday, November 26, 2003

Long time no entry. I just got out of the hospital after nearly a month's stay. I'm 14 weeks pregnant and at home on hyperalimentation, aka total parenteral nutrition (TPN) via PICC number three.

My trusted doctor of several years dropped me because my case was getting too complicated, and he doesn't have medical malpractice insurance. I was devastated. I tried to get on with other doctors but they either didn't accept my insurance or didn't accept anyone as sick as I am. My former doctor's partner referred me to the same doctors who mistreated and neglected me in the first horrific pregnancy. I absolutely refused and felt abandoned and lost. I ended up basically picking a name out of a phone book, but that experienced doctor didn't have time to see me. Instead I got the 34-year-old whippersnapper fresh out of residency. I lamented this "curse," but it was the best thing that ever happened to me.

He is taking super care of me and Tummy Lumpkin (TL). Matria called me one morning, and evidently, I didn't sound "right" to the nurse. She got me in to see the doctor right away. He examined me, put me in the hospital, and prescribed TPN. My nutrition was plummeting. For example, normal albumin (protein) levels are supposed to be around 22 and I was at 2. I haven't eaten anything in several weeks, but the TPN is keeping me alive.

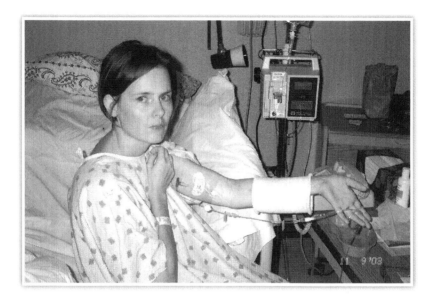

PICC 3: Holding nicely! The fabric on my arm is actually one of Hubby's tube socks with the ends cut off. These things make *great*, protective PICC covers. I slid it down so you could see the PICC. On my arm you can see the plastic sticker which is actually a clip that helps to prevent the line from pulling out of the site even a smidge. This is a PICC done right, folks! I love it so much I would marry it!

Let's take a moment to talk about attractive OBs. *No one wants this.* Well, no one who is too sick to wax her legs, pluck her brows, shave her pits, brush her teeth or bathe regularly. It's intimidating to be so gnarly around one who does not possess wrinkles and jowls and maybe even a merciful facial malignancy. What I wouldn't give for a doc with a bulbous nose or a crooked smile right about now. For the seriously ill patient only a crusty, old, unattractive OB will really do. We're talking about a doctor of Walter Matthau proportions. But no, I had to get the Keanu Reeves of OBs, and yes, my gastroenterologist asked him to perform a *rectal,* which he did, much to my humiliation.

That's the way it goes.

In the hospital I was having some problems like fevers, funky liver enzyme levels and gallbladder problems. I've got sludge (gut mud made out of tiny bile stones), and I may or may not need to get the gallbladder removed before this is all over. That's no big deal. The liver stuff is pretty important. If I get fatty infiltration of the liver, for example, that's not good. I could croak or something, so they have adjusted my TPN-related lipids.

During my stay I started sipping melted ice. I can get down about a half a cup of water a day this way. I am **ELATED** about this! Something goes down my throat and into my stomach! It makes me feel a little normal.

FYI, if you have suffered some devastation or another and are in the hospital with your face smashed in and your brain in a jar by the bed, every one of the hospital staff who enters your room will ask, "How are you doing today?"

For the first week I just sort of gave them a puzzled look and said, "Hanging in there." After nearly a month of this it got on my nerves and this is how it went:

Them: How are you doing today?

Me: I'm eating through a tube, and you?

And the award for the most asinine comment goes to a nurse who asked me:

"Well, have you *tried* eating a sandwich?"

I felt like saying, "Nah, it's just too much fun risking my life to eat through this tube."

Nuts.

Before I got admitted to the hospital I finally found a home health care nurse that *rocks*. When I got admitted her supervisor started coming to visit me in the hospital on a regular basis. This man was grieving from a recent miscarriage that he and his wife had suffered. Much of his conversation involved miscarriage, and while he was friendly, he made the well-meaning comment, "You're lying here *about to lose your baby*, and people shouldn't be stressing you out." For whatever reason, this really got to me. I am fighting HG with everything I have, and I need people to stay rational around me. I don't demand that people tell me only positive things, but I do want people to be reasonable. Things are rough, but there are no signs that I'm about to lose my baby. Severe HG is a seriously sucky situation, but people fight like heck and can still come out of it with living children. I know this poor guy is viewing life through the lens of a painful miscarriage right now and that this is probably his way of working it out, but I'm not a trained therapist, and it took a lot of energy to be there for him during these long conversations. It was also depressing for me to constantly talk about prenatal death when I'm trying to focus on prenatal survival and getting through each day. For my health, for my baby, I want to move in positive directions when I can.

I never meant to tattle on this guy. I endured it for so long, because I know the value of a good home health care nurse, and I was paranoid that I might lose her if this man didn't like me. But my favorite hospital nurse came in after his last visit and caught me crying. She had just seen this man walk out the door and knew something must have happened, so she inquired, and I confessed. She bolted out the door before I could finish, caught the man at the elevator, and told him he was never again to speak to me about miscarriage or losing my baby. She informed him that I was in my room crying because of him, and it wasn't good for me or the baby.

An hour or so later I received a call from my rockin' home health care nurse. She sounded odd, and she told me that she could no longer be my nurse when I got home. I asked why, and she told me, very carefully, that after his visit with me her supervisor called a sudden meeting and recommended that I was simply too sick to be managed by their company. She was terribly sorry but told me that was all she could say. She has a little boy to take care of; she values her job.

You think this sort of thing can't happen, because in a world of adults and professionals it's not supposed to. But guess what. It did. So I had to find a different local company to send out yet another new nurse, and I have to watch her like a hawk in case she doesn't really know what she is doing like so many before her. There is no science to this. You get what you get. And sometimes self-advocacy really can shoot you in the foot.

On a positive note, I got to hear TL's heartbeat several times in the hospital. Got good pictures too. One picture was taken at 12 weeks, 4 days or so, and you can see TL's hand clearly. You can count all five fingers.

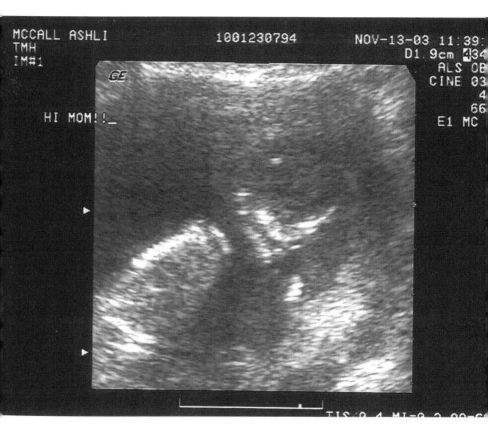

Five fingers!

The hospital sonographer said she has seen 9-week-old twins batting the yolk sac back and forth like a balloon. She also sees little 14-week-old boys holding their danglies. It starts in the womb, ladies. Doc says I can get one of GE's new 4D sonograms if we can make it to around 30 or so weeks. I'll post that too.

This new OB is having a hard time getting information from the old one who wants nothing to do with any of this (liability and apathy). For this reason, the new doc is watching the cervix closely before just automatically doing a cerclage for the incompetent cervix issue. This means pelvics galore.

Any type of "spelunking" is not good for a gal with my issues. I'm approaching the 15th week, and that week is always emotionally difficult, considering the fact that in my first pregnancy my very-much-wanted child died in an HG-related termination.

Well, I'm feeling pretty bad right about now, so I need to get back to my prison cell. Lots to do today. I need to change my Zofran site, so I'm going to be pulling a tiny catheter out of one leg and then shoving another one in the other leg via needle. After that it will be time for me to lance a finger for the hundredth time to check my blood glucose level (a must when on TPN). If it's too high I will jab myself with two units of insulin. If it's too low I will know it, because I will see dead relatives floating around the light at the end of the tunnel. D'har.

Actually, I bottomed out in the hospital because they were giving me too much insulin, and baby, it was freaky. I couldn't breathe, I was sweating, my heart was racing and my body initiated a POWERFUL sugar craving. And even though I'm still not able to eat, I would have donated a kidney for a mini Snickers bar.

On top of all this, I have to take my temperature, check my ketones, and phone in a bunch of info about pump totals and junk like that. This is all stuff I'd be too lazy to do if I was healthy, forget about being sick!

Quick update on husband: He's stressed being a "single" parent. He is hanging in there however. He is annoying me like crazy with all his complaints, but I couldn't do this without him, and I know he is taxed with so very much responsibility to carry alone.

Quick update on son: He goes to Pre-K where he is sometimes bored out of his skull. When our homeschooling was interrupted, we were learning world geography, and he was half-way through Kindergarten math. His Pre-K class however was learning their colors. And we're supposed to expect the kid not to have behavior problems? Plus, he takes after me, so naturally he's going to be a stubborn butt. I fail to see the problem.

The teacher has demanded that he be evaluated (aka diagnosed with something) by a psychologist. Meanwhile she was not fulfilling her end of the agreement to send home daily reports. We wanted to change his diet as well, but she gave us a week to see results. Ugh.

Anyway, she wants that "evaluation" and she will get it, because it's a private school, and they can kick your kid out for sneezing, while you still have to foot the entire bill. If we are seen as uncooperative it may not be good, and this is literally a day care situation. We are in a bit of a fix with that.

My son will get his big fat ADHD label, we will steadfastly refuse to medicate him and somehow all will be so much better than if the teacher had just given us some real time for the dietary alterations to kick in. To her credit, she is now doing well with the daily reports (after being called on it). Ugh. Ugh.

I have also noticed some of the results of being socialized by other children all day long. My son has begun to feel unsure about himself and his choices. At Show & Tell he wanted to bring in a fetal model to show how big his sibling was, but after a while he worried that the other kids would tease him. HE IS FOUR! It was letter "B" week and some other kid ended up bringing in a baby doll and no one made fun. When my son learned that it was OK to bring in a baby he wanted to bring in the model. Now we have to wait until "F" week for "fetus." Great.

I can't be there for him. The whole thing is depressing.

I missed Reformation Day (fake Halloween for Christians who dig Martin Luther), will miss Thanksgiving (unless they figure out a way to add turkey to my TPN) and will miss my son's birthday party. NOW THAT IS ROUGH!!! He's turning five and I'm not able to go to the party! Waaaaaaaaaaaaaa! **HG SUCKS!**

This is the update. We are still alive. I would never have been able to make it even this far without God. *Never.* We would have been done for long ago.

Thank you for all your earnest prayers. He hears you. Please keep it up. I *really* like eggnog, and wouldn't mind being able to drink some at Christmas. He can raise the dead, people, so I think I have a pretty good shot at this eggnog thing.

P.S.
One thing I forgot to mention. This pregnancy has thus far cost my insurance company over $60,000 (and I'm only 14 weeks). They have a contracted deal where they don't have to pay as much as it would normally cost, so I doubt they have actually

spent the above amount. Still, I'm racking up red points for them, and they no likey.

At no time did my health care professionals ever suggest termination to me. My current doctor has only ever worked diligently to afford me every available, positive option. He is even ready to put me on corticosteroids at week 16 as I requested. Everyone is aware that the goal is to fight HG and have a living child. While running up astronomical medical bills in the hospital however, my HMO caseworker, the same one who prevented me from getting a mechanical pump with my first PICC line, called to make sure I "knew" that I had the option to terminate the pregnancy. I told her I'd sooner die. I should have hung up on her instead. I think it's disgusting how the HMO would prey on a woman who has endured months of severe suffering with months to go. I can imagine other women thinking, "You know, this could all be over in five minutes. Hmmm." Actually, I *don't* have to imagine. I've been there, done that, *hated* it. It is not the answer.

Winston Churchill said "Give us the tools and we'll finish the job." Well, amen. HG moms need care, not despair. I'm glad that this time I knew the difference.

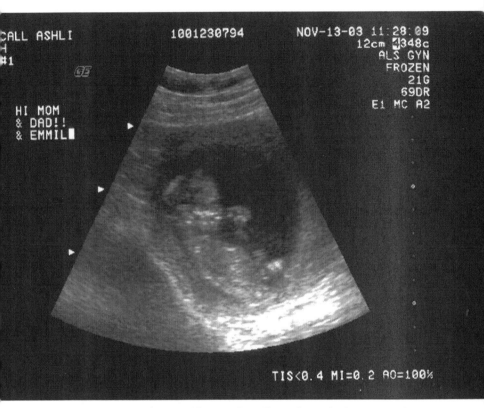

TL sucking thumb at 12 weeks. Our first baby was three weeks older when sadly, due solely to HG, we aborted.

December

Wednesday, December 10, 2003

I am delivering my update from the hospital where I was sent roughly five seconds after my last update. It happened the day after Thanksgiving to be exact. My husband came into the bedroom annoyed asking, "Why are you moaning? Does it make you feel better?" Funny, I hadn't realized I was moaning. The more I thought about it, I was not only moaning but twisting the sheets.

When I have the flu I twist the sheets. My ankles nearly screw themselves off as my legs writhe all over the mattress. My arms and shoulders practice unending jerky movements, a sort of pseudo chorea. All of these things were present. In addition, I was freezing while dripping bullets of sweat. I took my temperature. Bingo. Fever. This is not a good sign on a PICC.

When my thermometer read 101 it was time to call my doctor who naively gave me his pager number, God bless him.

"You know what this means."

(I do?)

"You have to come back to the hospital."

I hung up and prepared to leave when I got another phone call. A family member was killed in a car wreck early that morning. He was his mother's only child, and now she wanted to die. A surreal, devastating blow.

By the time I got off the phone and pulled into the hospital parking lot I had a temperature of 103 and was puking up blood. This was no streaky emesis. It was bold, fresh, solid-red puke that quickly turned brown when mixed with bile and gastric acids. Scary puke.

"You know what this means." started Dr. Keanu.

I must confess I'm never totally sure what anything means, but when he starts with that sentence I know it's nothing good.

"We have to pull the PICC."

And pull it they did. Then they hooked me up to a peripheral (regular IV) for fluids and antibiotics. Pee tests confirmed that I had one heck of a nasty bladder infection. It was so nasty in fact that the doctor half doubted that I'd done it correctly.

"We should have put a catheter in to test it," he said, "but I didn't want to torture you."

This from a man who stuck his finger up my butt.

In addition to the bladder infection the PICC grew staph when the tip was cultured. I.e., the PICC appeared to be infected too.

Antibiotics.

The second day in the hospital I still felt like death. While my nurse was changing my sheets I sat there puking, peeing and having glycerin diarrhea all over myself in a chair. She stood me up, and I told her I was going to pass out if I didn't sit back down. After being told that there was "no physical reason" why I would be passing out (what?!) I crawled into the bed. The nurse stood over me annoyed with my "behavior" before finally shaking her head in genuine disgust.

"Ashli, Ashli, Ashli," she stated with disdain, "Pregnancy is a normal part of life."

I was completely dumbfounded.

"Do you think I am doing this to myself?!?" I asked incredulously.

"I didn't say that," she said. "I just think you're getting yourself all worked up."

Holy smokes, people! She takes the cake. She stomps all over the sandwich nurse. She wins the Pulitzer of unbelievably asinine comments. On day three I began to feel like a human being again. I got rid of the nurse.

How do you solve a problem like starvation? Put in another PICC of course. That's right. Number four. It is the biggest PICC I've had and was a major pain to get in. The IV therapist shoved and shoved this thing up my vein, but it kept crimping.

"What's happening?" I wanted to know.

The reply: "The introducer is hanging on some kind of nerve or tissue or something."

"Some kind of nerve or tissue or something." These words in this succession—well, let's just say it's not the kind of thing that relaxes you and helps you get a 4 French tube up your arm, around your shoulder and into your chest. No siree.

At that particular moment, even the rectal started to look good in comparison. He leaned on my left arm, forced the confounded line in, and by golly, it finally took. One X-ray later the placement was confirmed and TPN was once again started. Personally, I think it's a little too far into the vein and possibly is pressing on the heart valve or something, because when I lie on my left side I have a tendency now to get heart palpitations. Weird ones too.

They feel kind of...deep. But at least for now I'm not telling my doctor, because you know what that means.

Back in my room I lay in bed thinking about the events and my poor Martha, the mother who had just lost her precious son in a car wreck. Soon I began to hear wailing in the hall outside my door. Wailing, wailing on. I couldn't integrate it until the words became loud and intelligible.

"Oh God, he was purple! My baby came out purple! Please God, I want my baby back! My baby's gone! My baby's gone!"

A stillborn son at 38 weeks.

A picture of Martha, thoroughly medically sedated and crouched in the corner of her hotel room, superimposed the event across the hall, and at once I heard these mothers wailing in tandem. An image of a world of wailing mothers lanced for a moment my safe bubble of sanity allowing the infection of death and grief to penetrate. I pressed my ear to the door willing compassion to be felt through the wood, through the hall, through the heart of this wounded, wounded soul.

"My baby! Purple and dead, please God, please! I want my baby back!"

I slid to the floor and cried. Ambling back into bed I couldn't help but wonder if I would revisit the freshness of such grief in my own life. Would this child I carry make it or be born purple and dead too?

But I have today, and today s/he is kicking quite plainly. This is my treasure. I will keep today no matter what. I'm 16 weeks on Monday, and they're trying to figure out what to do with me.

I need to stay here longer if I'm going to start steroids. But hey, I've got a blog and a laptop; It doesn't matter how long I stay!

Husband update: He's being nicer because he's less stressed not having to raise a child single-handedly *and* play nurse to me at home.

Son update: He had his fifth birthday at a kiddie pizza place. The woman assigned to his party table (I like to call them "Chuck E. Wenches") was dancing and getting the birthday boy to do what she was doing. "Swing left, swing right, now jump!" She began to jump, and he just stood there like a deer caught in the headlights. Literally. On the video tape I could see the objects of his mesmerization: the Chuck E. Wenche's perky, bouncing boobs. Oblivious she cried, "Jump! Jump!" In a mad birthday frenzy the new five-year-old bounded into the air, lunged forward, and cupped both tiny meat hooks around fistfuls of firm, ripe university flesh.

"AAAiiiieeee!" cried the Chuck E. Wench as she crossed a shield of arms over her violated anatomy. The look on my kid's face asked, "Did I just do that?" For a moment he was shocked. I thought he might cry, but instead he hid his mouth in his hand and giggled.

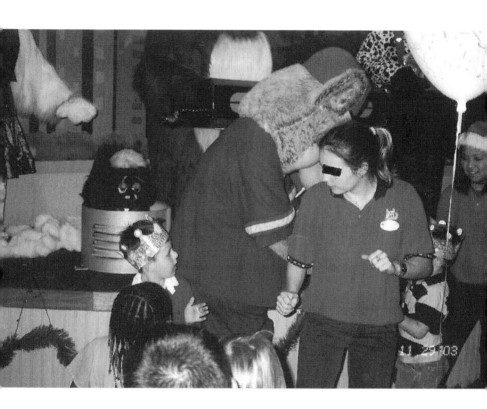

I hope all of you are doing better than I am. I'm a little bummed, because I lost the picture of my fourth PICC line, which I had intended to use to horrify you. But horrifying people is an art and takes a certain degree of health to fully master, so perhaps I'll find it and proceed when I'm feeling better.

In the mean time I'm going to sit here in the hospital while all my healthy caretakers continuously horrify *me* with their in, out, up and down procedures, and comments like "You know what this means," dance like arsenic sugarplums in the hollow of my puking gourd.

Monday, December 15, 2003

Hello all. I am 17 weeks today and EATING!!! Albeit only certain things yet THINGS no less! To me, this is Christ feeding 5,000+ with two fish and five loaves of bread: a miracle. Often we overlook life's wonderments as we shake our fists at the sky demanding that God prove Himself. We are fools.

I am drinking ginger ale, Sprite and grape Ginseng-Up, and eating things like soup, fresh fruit, bread, small salads, scrambled eggs, and even a *7-ounce filet mignon!* (Thank you, Uncle Garry!) I am no longer on the Zofran pump, so perhaps it's the steroids. Time and steroids.

"When I'm not busy peeing on myself while puking my head off and starving, I like to play professional football. That's why I take 'Roids."

But I have to start tapering the corticosteroids this week, and I'm a little anxious. I **do not** want to slip back even one tiny little step. If I never vomit again in all my life it will be far too soon.

Last week's sonogram revealed a gall bladder which is still full of sludge. The sonographer graciously, sneakily gave me some pictures of the baby to encourage me and remind me of the little person I am fighting for. Back out in the hallway, waiting for the friendly tech from my floor to come take me (and my pole) back to my room, a woman waiting for her sonogram asked me how far along I was. She was 13 weeks and we chatted for a moment. I noticed that her hair was as ratty and gross as mine, and she looked like a heroin addict. Of course I knew.

"You've got hyperemesis, don't you?" I asked.

"Yep," she nodded.

Insta-friends.

We talk on the phone daily, encouraging each other when nurses are mean or weekend docs on call are clueless. We commiserate.

"Thank God you understand how I feel," she once told me.

We are a tiny little pocket of women who are devastated by an illness that barely anyone understands, validates, or even knows exists.

"There were times when I just felt I couldn't go on, couldn't do it anymore," she lamented.

Oh, how I understand.

"I brushed my teeth today!" she gushed.

No small triumph. It is a blessing that we have been able to connect this way.

Perhaps I will come off the TPN today. They have been tapering me down as I have been able to eat more. I'm a little anxious of course. When I'm finally feeling half-way human I don't want to mess with anything. But I have to get rid of this PICC. Once they take me off the TPN I'll keep the PICC until my health has been established, i.e., until I can maintain an adequate daily caloric intake. The lumens (capped tube access which some might call "ports") will have to be flushed with saline and heparin every 12 hours for two weeks, and, if all is well, then I can get the PICC removed.

I would truly like to be home for Christmas.

After this half of the ordeal is over, for the remainder of the pregnancy I will still be on bed rest for the incompetent cervix. I go for another check up in a week.

Heard Pumpkin Butt's heartbeat this morning and am feeling all sorts of wonderful movements. "Mother, I'm here. Love me today!"

And I am finally physically healthy enough to do so.

Tuesday, December 16, 2003

They took me off the TPN last night and the nausea level doubled. This is still not a tragedy since my level has been down to a two on a scale of 1-10. So for all you mathematically challenged folks out there, I'm on a level four. Living at level four consists of feeling yucky all day and woozy when food comes around. I'll think, "Oy, I can't eat that," but I'll try, and it will go down without immediately flying out of my throat and nostrils. In fact, at level four you can keep things down. *I haven't thrown up in over a week*, people! Prayers for eggnog!

Let's talk about Poopbutt. This child is rolling around in there like someone set up a trampoline. It is delightful! Somersaults and all. You can even feel movement from the outside now. It's amazing. And disturbing how people can think that's nothing in there. It's not nothing. Anyone who has carried a kicking child knows that. Kick, kick, roll! My heart sings. It **sings**!

"Love me, Mama!"

I do, little Kicky-pher!

And then the rushing sorrow sets in for the first child. Oh, the first child...

My lungs fill with fluid sadness. I drown a little, die a little, dumb with the contradiction and horror of what I have done. The miracle life of this new child connects me to the first. What am I to say? That this is a real child but that one wasn't? Fantasies are convenient but unconvincing. Life is a sequence of progression, a kind of Newtonian law, moving in a straight line unless acted upon by an outside force. And what a destructive force it was. In this there are no illusions nor mulligans. So there isn't anything to do but live through this moment like all the others. It's a complicated, impossible wound that all apologies will never heal.

Whir. Click. Survival Mode: Insert abrupt change of subject.

No TPN. Wow. No tubing and pole. All day I have been fumbling for a phantom tube as I exit the bed for the pee-measuring top hat in the bathroom. No tube! Freedom! Get it through your head! It has been months since I've had no kind of tube. I don't know what to do with myself. Of course, I still have two unsightly lumens hanging out of my arm making me look like a cyborg. I still can't take a shower. "We'll cover them up," they say. Indeed. I tried twice, and the apparatus is always soaked through. None for me, thanks.

Kickypher is kicking again. "Hello to all who read my mommy's diary! I am a real person with a real leg, and I can even kick with it!" My son says, "Bad baby! Don't kick my mama!" No amount of money in the world, people. No amount of money or status or success—nothing compares to these two little children of mine.

OK, share time.

I want to tell you of a woman I met yesterday. She came into my room because one of my nurses told her about me and thought I might be encouraged by a visit. This woman's son is in the neonatal intensive care unit. He is two pounds and was born at 25 weeks. His 44-year-old mama had placenta previa in the worst way. She was losing blood faster than they could put it in her and had been in the hospital for six weeks passing grapefruit sized clots and just buckets of blood.

The placenta metastasized. She thought she was having the baby one night and passed a clot the size of a baby. The doctor said it was time to deliver. The woman lost too much blood and had zero blood pressure. She rolled her eyes back into her head and out she went.

Immediately she saw a dark road. She calls it a tunnel but says it was more like a dark country road at night. She said that above this dark road there was a shining white light that was brighter than any light she had ever seen, brighter than the sun. She said she was not afraid at all but was filled with peace. She told me she doesn't know for sure but that she feels in her very being that the light was God.

The surgeons brought her back. They got the baby boy out and tried to save her life, but she wouldn't stop bleeding. They told her husband not to expect her to make it. She saw the road again and the light and felt total peace and contentment. She reiterated that it was the most peaceful feeling, and there was absolutely no fear. It was a light of comfort, a light of love, and she had a sense that this was her home, a place where she belonged. She trusted God to take care of her surviving children.

Her husband, preacher, and friends gathered in a circle outside of the operating room and prayed. Surgeons found the placenta growing behind her bladder. They had to cut her bladder in half to get the placenta out and then repair the bladder. The bleeding stopped and the light faded away. She came to, and they told her she had a baby boy.

All of this happened last month. Now she comes to visit her struggling son every day, and there are always problems. Right now he has air in his intestines and is backing up. They are doing the best they can to save him, but his mother has seen the Light and she is full of peace.

I tell you her story because she sat here in my room telling it to me. I am told that doctors and nurses have been talking about it for weeks, and I had been waiting anxiously to meet her.

I am not trying to impart any neat and tidy moral by sharing her story. It simply is what it is, and you will decide for yourself what it means. I only had to tell it.

Hubby and son have the puking/diarrhea bug. It is tenacious. Hubby has had it for four days now. He says he has gained new insight into my suffering. He said he spent one entire morning puking and having diarrhea. He knows that I spent entire months like that.

He said, "I don't know how you do it. I couldn't do it."

I was so grateful I wanted to cry. How soon he will forget though. I will ask him to run out and get me something to eat and he will say, "Oh sheesh, I'm tired, can't you just eat something that's already here?" And I will blow up and say, "Hello, I didn't eat or drink for 11 weeks. 11 WEEKS!!! Now go get me some beans and weenies like I asked you to, confound it!!!"

I am terrified to go home. I do not want to catch this stuff. **Terrified**, I say! Begging the doctors to keep me here. I would like to go home Friday at the soonest. Unfortunately, it doesn't always work that way. The HMO however, would be stupid to want to get me out of here three days early so it could pay for two more weeks. They'd better think long and hard about that, horses' rears that they are. Oh, just wait until I get out of this fix and everything is paid for. That HMO representative is going to be sorry that she called me in my hospital room and harassed me with the "suggestion" of abortion.

Wednesday, December 17, 2003

Today is a day for being grateful. I woke up this morning in tears so thankful for the health and blessings that God has given me. In the midst of so much suffering, I have learned a vast amount. This isn't to say that once life goes on I won't be an ungrateful idiot again, but I hope this experience keeps my sleepy eyes open at least a miracle-registering slit. I don't want life to be lost on me.

I thanked my doctor this morning from the bottom of my heart. I wept as I expressed my gratitude. He didn't know what to do with it really. "Just say 'You're welcome,' and get out!" I told him. I wept as I thanked my tech and my favorite nurses. Grateful, grateful. One of my nurses said my doctor commented that I was "emotional" this morning. "It's probably the prednisone," she reminded him. Oh, if they only knew! Few short weeks ago I prayed to die, and now I am praying to live and love. How can I not weep?

I told one of my nurses how funny it was that when you give your heart to some people they don't really know what to do with it. She told me it's because no one ever gives their heart anymore. She said it's rare that people even say thank you. I've seen them though, while I've been here. Really thankful people. A few of them.

One of my grey-haired doctors immediately turned into a speechless 17-year-old when I told him how sincerely grateful I was to him. I found it quite charming and funny the same. I don't do it to make people feel out of sorts or to amuse myself with their discomfort, but it is so odd to me, the nature of man and his inability to freely love. Children are not this way. Adults learn it after years of rejection. Should I feel inappropriate for failing to observe mature emotional convention? My rescuers dug me out of a deep hole that stank of death. I could kiss them all through a thousand grateful tears!

"Never let loyalty and kindness get away from you! Wear them like a necklace; write them deep within your heart. Then you will find favor with both God and people, and you will gain a good reputation." Proverbs 3:3-4

Someone from dietary (the kitchen downstairs) put a guardian angel pin on my tray today. My tech says she has never met a patient like me. We are planning to BBQ once all is well many moons from now. I have made many special pals here in the hospital, and so you see that while I did not wear kindness and loyalty like a necklace to gain a good reputation, it happened anyway, which only goes to show that God knows what He's talking about. "Preach on, Sister." I can't help it.

"Has the LORD redeemed you? Then speak out. Tell others he has saved you from your enemies." Psalms 107:2

Sometimes my biggest enemy is myself. Look back at my termination posts this pregnancy. I can honestly say that the Lord saved me (and my baby) from myself. This is no small miracle. I will talk more about that tomorrow when I share with you two notes that I wrote myself during a pivotal point.

Tomorrow! I get out! I go to stay with my mother-in-law. She loves me when I'm pregnant! I should stay this way all the time! HA!

Squirmy is squirming. "Hi, peoples! Pray for my mommy and me!"

:-)

Saturday, December 20, 2003

Hey, guys. Sorry about dropping off the face of the earth. I'm not going to post those two notes right now, because my time is limited.

Update: I got booted out of the hospital on Wednesday night. The HMO came in and began harassing me throughout the day. They were pretty ugly. I ended up going to my in-laws (where I am now), because the hubby has had the puking/diarrhea bug. They have been taking good care of me.

Tapering the steroids is a little difficult. I feel pretty yucky as the levels go down. And from being on TPN for so long the ol' gastrointestinal tract kind of went dormant. It is having quite a time waking back up. Not helping at all is the cervical issue that keeps me mired to the bed. Can't digest anything or even pass gas when I'm lying down all day long. Ugh.

Good news: Yesterday we got the "fetal anatomy study" done. After all of these multiple drugs/treatments/ailments/etc., the baby is perfect in every way, praise God. Not only that but...

SHE'S A GIRL!

Thanks for all the prayers. Please keep them up.

Would like everyone to know that I had a glass of *eggnog* the other day! It wasn't as good as I remembered. Probably because I still feel like poop.

Overheard someone talking on the phone: "We know what the baby is going to be. It's going to be a little girl."

How do we know "it's" *going to be* a little girl? Because we saw a little baby giney (labia, the works). Don't you kind of already have to **be** a girl to have a vagina? I mean, turnips don't have vaginas. She's not a turnip. The child is a child, is a girl, is a she, not an it. I know I'm defensive. I'm grappling with what happened and the humanity of gestating children. I feel like Charlton Heston trying to convince the world that Soylent Green is people, and no one will listen.

But if you can hear me, I want you to know that what is in my womb is a human child, a baby. And the baby is a girl, our daughter, Elise, which means "God's oath." And furthermore, I am her mother, not her "mother-to-be." What is all this work I've been doing if not motherhood? I haven't just been sitting here contemplating my navel!

A girl...a **GIRL!**

All of this is miraculous. Every moment is God in action. He is alive and very well, and the music of my heart sings His name!

Monday, December 22, 2003

Oh boy. Bed rest. Already I've become an ingrate. Pathetic.
I remember a time not too long ago when I would have chopped
off my legs just to be able to eat, without the slightest concern
for bed rest. But now I am eating and on bed rest, and all of a
sudden just eating doesn't seem good enough, no. I want to be
able to vacuum the floor and make dinner. Not gonna happen.
Bed rest, Cervix Girl. Get it through your melon! Mmmm,
melon.

The wonderful people at my local organic co-op have been
pampering me by picking up, sorting out, and delivering produce/
dairy. Today we got watermelon, Sharlyn melons, Fuji apples, Pink
Lady apples, tangerines, oranges, Red Bartlett pears, etc. Gonna
be a feast, boys and girls. My favorite in the delivery today is
something I've been dreaming about for a while now: fresh
delicious beets with tops. Mmm! Steam the little devils, tops
and all. Butter and salt, and give me a call! Good luck, hubby. I'm
slightly afraid to eat them because for a day or so I will not be
able to monitor cervical clues well. Beets, for those who don't
know, cause the urine to turn pink and sometimes nearly red.
Same goes for the stool. I remember the first time I ate a big
bunch. I went to the bathroom and thought I was hemorrhaging.
Pretty funny. Beeeeeets!

By the way, I'm drinking eggnog as we speak!

Alright, alright, the bay-girl:

Elise is moving all the time. She is a mess! She comforts me
though, because every time I wake up in the night and don't feel
her moving she wakes up for me and gives me a jab. Already
taking care of me. My poor dove. During the sonogram we

could see a perfect profile of her face. Her nose and lips—everything. She was moving constantly. Her little mouth was sucking and sucking as she waved her hand in front of it trying to get that thumb in. My kids are not coordinated, but they get their passion for nourishment from me, I can tell you. The 4D sonogram is going to be really neat. I think I may wait until 26 weeks to get it. The later the better I hear.

OK, now for the heavy, depressing part of this entry:

A few days ago I told you about two notes that I wrote myself early in the pregnancy when things were really going from bad to much worse. I know I can sit here and say, "Folks, it was really bad, so bad," but if you haven't been there, you just can't imagine. I'm not criticizing. I know it's this way for all of us. The first time I heard the story of Jesus fasting for 40 days and nights, I quickly thought, "Gee, that would suck," but that was the extent of my personal investment. I couldn't understand even if I tried. But this pregnancy, I went almost twice as long without eating (though I had a feeding tube), and I didn't even choose to do it. Because of this, I now have a better appreciation of Christ's fast than I ever did before. My point is, I'm not sure that you will understand or even be able to forgive the words that you are about to read. Luckily, you are not my judge. However, for what it's worth, I invite you into the dark arena of my blackest heart to learn more about HG, to witness the bleak moments of human despair that can only lead to death and more despair, and then to experience the hope that rescued me and my baby girl.

I was six weeks pregnant and in the hospital for the first or second admission. I knew it was only the beginning. I was sick to my core and terrified of living one more day like that. The living death. The rack. Torture. I wanted out. I began to think like an animal, to make plans I knew I would regret. I knew the sick Ashli and the healthy Ashli were two totally different people, and I had to be convinced that the plans I was making were necessary. But were they? I wanted each point of view to present her case before I passed final judgment. I also wanted an emotional snapshot of where I was when the die was cast. And so I wrote two notes to myself:

Note to Healthy Ashli (from Sick Ashli):
"If you are reading this then you opted for another therapeutic termination. This is unbelievable and yet understandable. I know how sad it is, but I want you to remember and cling to two very important things: 1) No matter what you tell yourself later on, there is *no way* you can live like this for 14 more weeks, and 2) the baby is as big as a grain of rice. This is the early first trimester; the child will not feel pain. I know you will pour over this pre-death note a million times wishing you had not done it, but you will be well then and not sick like you are now. Terminating again was wrong. Yes. No denial here. The illness was too much to bear, and you were not as faithful and strong as you wanted to be. While the baby was from God, the illness was not; it's a conflict that will be hard to resolve. And the fact that the baby is due in your birth month will only twist the knife; your own birthday will become even more complicated. But the current pain and anxiety are such that one more day and 14 more weeks of this are more immediately pressing. Even from here, I can see that it isn't really justifiable, but who can attend distant concerns in the face of a pulverizing present? You will have to *cling for dear life* to the facts that the unaware baby felt no pain and you honestly could not take 14 more weeks of this. This rationale will be all you have, so you had better find a way to value it above all else. And you must never attempt a pregnancy again."

How many lies could you pick out? I should hold a raffle and give away jellybeans to the person who can count that high.

My dear abortion-supporting friend who used to work at Planned Parenthood, and who almost terminated her daughter over HG, came to the hospital and told me that if I ended the pregnancy she was certain I would kill myself or lose my mind and that either way my son would have no mother.

Before we even knew the sex, my husband kept telling me this was our baby girl promised from God and that termination was not an option.

My pastor told me that everything I was feeling, thinking and planning was absolutely understandable, quite normal and rational—but that I must not do it. He reminded me that I knew how God felt about it and that it was against the laws He put into place because He is holy and because God practices strange math: the fetters of His laws are freeing and give me the best chance at a happy life. My pastor was sensitive and bold, and he supported me by saying **NO.**

And what of God's support? Must the obvious be said? He gave me the sacrificial suffering of His Son for my example and His very Word, which is always there to speak if I will but listen.

The shoulder angel of me wrote her own letter in response to the one with which my shoulder devil tempted me:

"Dear Ashli,
Don't you dare take such advice. It is the siren song of death. The Lord your God is with you, and the life of this child is His to direct. The LORD has rescued you both by providing necessary treatments. Pray that His guiding, saving hand continues. And praise His glorious name, for He is your salvation and is inspiring you to know something of love through courageous acts of personal surrender. You shall neither be demonized nor separated from your child if you keep your heart full of the Lord

Who has spoken to you already through the Word and through the hearts of other believers whom He has sent. So be not afraid, for God is your strength, your shield. Trust in Him with all your heart, and you will be helped. Do not kill your child. God is with you both, and you can do all things with Christ. You can suffer as greatly as you think you can't. May God forgive you for hopeless thoughts during desperate times. He has suffered and prevailed; He has paved the way. Hold fast to your faith and be blessed."

Now, don't think I don't know how weird these "multiple personality" writings are. They will seem even weirder to you unless you have been held hostage by such an illness or situation. Just remember that Tom Hanks' character in Cast Away started cracking up too: The man was talking to a volleyball. I needed a way to give audience to the different facets of myself that were coming out under immense duress and guiding decisions. A writing exercise seemed appropriate.

Decide what you think about those facets of me: desperation and hope. One filled with terror and selfishness and the other filled with thoughts of God and something better than even my own life. One would have killed my daughter, disappointed God, and ruined me for good. The other got us this far.

My child was promised to me. I know it because I have her today. Perhaps tomorrow will never come, but I live this moment for and in the promise. She is God's oath, my Elise, and it's only because of Him that we are still together.

Wednesday, December 24, 2003

Mad cow disease found in the U.S.? Great. I just had a big pot of chili last night and have been craving beef like a bovine-eating lunatic. Sheesh.

I forgot to tell you guys:

When I was getting my fanny booted out of the hospital there was a PICC issue. I had been registering tiny fevers for a couple of days, and my in-laws were pretty freaked out about keeping my lumens patent (flushing them). The lumens were too short for me to reach with one hand. I couldn't screw the hypodermics on, and my in-laws were just terrified to touch them due to the fact that the line was just outside the opening of my heart and due to the former staph infection. I talked to Dr. Keanu about it, and he just broke down and said, "Let's pull the line." I was supposed to have the thing until after Christmas, but he pulled it.

Two days later I took my first real shower in three months. I had to sit down in the middle of it, because it was so exhausting. I can't stand up for too long without getting shaky and breathless. I've also got tachycardia. I've literally got the pulse of a three-year-old. I'm getting moon-faced from the steroids and from generally stuffing my face without being able to exercise one calorie away. However, I prefer to blame it on the 'roids, because it implies that all I have to do to stop looking like Jabba the Hut is stop taking a pill.

Wella, wella. Happy Christmas Eve, people. Remember the Reason for the season.

Picture Linus with his blue blanket shepherd's hat:

"And there were shepherds living out in the fields nearby, keeping watch over their flocks at night. An angel of the Lord appeared to them, and the glory of the Lord shone around them, and they were terrified. But the angel said to them, 'Do not be afraid. I bring you good news of great joy that will be for all the people. Today in the town of David a Savior has been born to you; He is Christ the Lord. This will be a sign to you: You will find a Baby wrapped in cloths and lying in a manger.'" Luke 2:8-12

Can they even *play* the Charlie Brown Christmas special on TV anymore? Or has the ACLU nipped that one in the bud too?

GOOD GRIEF.

Saturday, December 27, 2003

Friendly advice: Make sure you have a cell phone or a phone card or something if you are ever admitted to the hospital.

As you will recall, I was readmitted when a family member died in a car wreck. We were both admitted to the same hospital the same day, he to the morgue and I to the O.B. floor. His mother was and is, of course, devastated. I placed many calls to her from the hospital to make sure she was still breathing and to grieve with her. Sometimes I got her answering machine and hung up. Today I got a phone bill informing me that each of these one-minute hang-up calls cost me 10 dollars. An eight-minute phone call cost me nearly $20. And so on and so forth. And we thought the admission bills were going to be the most pressing financial issue! We called the bandits known as Sprint, and they informed me in their most compassionate, touching voice that I was straight out of luck, but happy New Year. I want their head on a platter, candied and spiral sliced for the holidays.

UGH.

Next month's bill is going to be merciless.

Elise has been inactive today. She has moved a few times but nothing like normal. Some cramping. I know I should be worried, but every time I try I just can't muster it. Isn't that odd?

Our neighbor brought over a tin of chocolate chip cookies. I have been carefully guarding the tin here in my Sealy Posturepedic lair. My husband came in and tried to get one, but the growling scared him away. There are three left. Mourn their passing.

I am swelling. Is it the cookies, the bed rest, the pregnancy or the drugs? I feel like something isn't quite right with my blood pressure. Malaise? Sort of, but not in the typical sense. I think it can wait until my next appointment. Famous last words.

I am going to try to get my doctor and my nefarious HMO to afford me some pneumatic compression cuffs. I am a double-risk for deep vein thrombosis and pulmonary embolism: I am pregnant and on bed rest. I think I still get a little dehydrated at times, which doesn't help. These cuff thingies are thigh-high and they have air pumped into them at differing intervals. This massages and compresses blood vessels in the legs significantly reducing the risk of blood clots and embolism. I don't imagine having difficulty getting Dr. Keanu to prescribe them. The insufferable HMO is yet another story.

Elise has decided to wake up for the writing of this diary entry. She is currently kickboxing for your entertainment. "Hi-YAA!"

The hubby has gone to get Chinese. I think this may be a grave mistake. The smell will probably kill me. I haven't had Chinese since the last diary entry about Chinese food in, what, September? Smells are getting worse again. Stomach's a little queasy. I thought I was going to throw up for the first time in ages last night, but it didn't happen. I am almost done tapering the 'roids. Four more days. I don't anticipate needing a PICC or going back to those days at this point. I think, for the most part, I will be OK. The issue for me is becoming the blood clots. I know I need not have issues, but I'd like to use my head and optimize my chances of success if I can. God does give us sense.

From the depths of her grieving Martha called the other day distraught and wanting to know what heaven was. I guess I haven't really thought about that so much. What would you have said? I said, finally, that it was home. At first I wondered if I'd muffed it, but the more I think about it, the more I am satisfied. Home. Yes. That has got to be it.

What did you get for Christmas? I got maternity/nursing clothes and Burt's Bees stuff. Money to cover hospital bills too. But not phone bills! Sprint! GRRRRR!

Last night my little boy came and snuggled in the bed with me. He fell asleep and proceeded to kick me in my back and kidneys all night long. From inside, Elise joined the kidney-kicking festivities in the wee small hours, and I was the happiest girl alive.

Monday, December 29, 2003

I have a sore throat. My eyes are dry and itchy. Oh yes, and I caught ringworm in the hospital. A nurse with cats? I now have a silver dollar sized splotch on my arm. Itchy, itchy. I was putting tea tree oil on it for a few days but then I started seeing internet warnings against it. Warnings without elaboration. Anyone out there know what the deal is on that? What does it supposedly do that can be harmful during pregnancy? Besides stink to high heaven.

Little Bit kicked so hard a couple of times this morning that she made me laugh! Boom. BOOM! She was pitching some kind of fit. She may have been asking for root beer, because when she got it she simmered down.

My beets are decaying in the veggie drawer. I haven't had the heart (or the nerve) to ask hubby to prepare them. I guess I'll have to pee pink some other time.

Someone from church made me a tray of coconut balls covered in chocolate. They go good with root beer. Little Bit will be born with rotten teeth and the shakes.

If I get one more Paris Hilton spam I'm going to have to hook back up to the Zofran pump. Yuck!

That Chinese food went down very well the other night. I am craving veggies lately. Probably due to the ringworm. Body, heal thyself! I think I should cut down on dairy, because of the calcium and the rumors that it helps to form blood clots. I'll ask Dr. Keanu, who will think I'm crazy.

I go for an appointment this week. I will ask lots of questions about nothing while pretending I am not actually on the receiving end of the pelvic he is sure to perform.

Wednesday, December 31, 2003

Went to the doctor's today. Dr. Keanu seemed genuinely encouraged by my overall wellbeing. I asked him about the pneumatic compression device, and after he was done laughing he informed me that it might be a tad on the overkill side. He said if I were using a bedpan then he might prescribe it. Then he scolded me about not doing my leg/foot exercises in bed, which I deserved. Then the pelvic came. I closed my eyes and thought about squirrels.

Squirrels in the yard.
Squirrels eating corn.
Squirrels climbing trees.
Squirrels, squirrels, not pelvics but squirrels!!!

Sigh...

He is going to watch my puffiness. Today is the last day of steroids, so the "swelling" should start going down a little or at least not get any worse. My husband told Dr. Keanu that he thought it had less to do with the pills and more to do with the truckloads of food I eat while lying in bed all day. Thank you, dear husband.

The walls in that office are shockingly thin. You can hear *everything* that is going on in the other rooms. My husband had me dying laughing while we were waiting for the doctor. I'm a loud laugher too. I get obnoxious; I snort and everything. I told him to knock it off or the baby would shoot out. He couldn't help himself. Everything was hilarious. That whole office must have thought we were lunatics. Dr. Keanu said he had another couple in today that reminded him of us. The woman is 36 weeks pregnant, and the husband got bored waiting for the doc, so he whipped out a magic marker and started drawing faces on his wife's big, pregnant belly. I want to meet this couple.

Before we went back to our exam room, the nurse gave us stickies upon which to write our questions. While we were waiting in the room I tried to get the hubby to give me a sticky. I was going to draw a big circle on it with a slash through it and stick it on my Underoos to ward off the pelvic. My husband said we weren't in high school.

We heard Stinkerbell's heartbeat. Nice and strong. Rapid thump-thumping, tiny and perfect. Human and alive. Someone's sister, granddaughter, cousin, niece, child...

Afterwards we got gyros. It is pronounced "year-ohs," but my husband says "Jie-rohs," which makes me giggle. They were gross. Lettuce is no longer agreeing with me. Just the thought of it makes me sick. I'd rather eat dirt. Or acorns. Or squirrels.

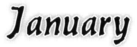

Friday, January 02, 2004

Bad news at the doctor's today. My cervix is shortening quickly. They want to do a cerclage here at 20 weeks. The cerclage could save Elise or kill her. If we choose not to do the cerclage that decision could save her or kill her. We don't know what to do.

This is all happening because of the bad choice I made in my first pregnancy, a choice I made due to HG. Bad choices have consequences. I am praying that God will intervene, but I understand that intervention can only happen if it is God's will. Please join me in praying for Elise's life. I want her to live here with us, and I want to grow old and have her outlive me.

I praise God for giving her to me and am so sorry that my misguided choice is threatening her life.

Even if she was only promised to me for a little while, I have had her this long and have very much enjoyed her life thus far. No matter what happens I have that. I will always have a daughter named Elise, and I will always love her. I am not sorry I fought for her with everything I had to give.

Even if she dies it has all been worth it.

Sunday, January 04, 2004

A very dear friend sent me an email today that prompted a response that I thought I'd share for those who are wondering how I am doing with the bad news and swiftly approaching decision:

"'The Lord is my strength and my shield; my heart trusts in Him, and I am helped.' Psalm 28:7

You couldn't know, but this was a very important scripture to me this pregnancy. When I was around six weeks pregnant I kept repeating it over and over again. It got me and Elise through some very rough times—times I thought would be impossible to get through.

The book of Job has been very guiding to me. I hope I am at the end of the story though! You know, the part where there's a happy ending and all is restored! But I read through Jesus' agony at Gethsemane and was reminded of the bitter cup. Christ did not particularly *want* to drink from that cup, but it was God's will, and so He did. Thus, I am reminded that this pregnancy may not end the way I want it to. I must submit and be willing even for Elise to die if that is what would bring the most honor and glory to the Lord Who knows and sees what I can't. Oh, but this is not an easy attitude!

I earnestly know that she may not live and that the Lord cannot be manipulated by good deed or attitude to save her if that is not His will. But perhaps He can be moved as He was moved by the people of Nineveh. Perhaps if He means for her to die He will take pity on my broken heart or will be moved by the prayers of others for her and will change His mind. I don't know. It's worrisome, I admit. Yet I know that even if everyone I love was lost from my life God would still be there. This has been the way of it. We are to love Him more than anyone, even our children. This is hard for me, but I think I am learning.

He is the Giver of life. How can anyone fault Him for assuming that which He Himself gave in the first place? How can one hate Him for giving the precious gift of even a moment of love? But we do it all the time! He is the Potter, and we are the clay. I have to remind myself and keep things in perspective. It is a constant battle for me. It does not come naturally or easily. God is teaching me many things. Above all, to borrow from C.S. Lewis, that He is not Who I say He is but who He knows Himself to be.

Anything inspiring or encouraging comes from the Holy Spirit and not me. I alone will only disappoint. It is a constant struggle to be less me and more of a person moved by the Holy Spirit.

I don't know what will become of Elise and me, but I know He loves us. All I can do now is beg for mercy for her life. What He does or does not do is His business, and I will always thank Him and praise Him for the miracle of my daughter no matter what."

Tuesday, January 06, 2004

I would like to thank all of you who are such a support during this very trying pregnancy. Some of you have brought me food, called me on the phone, emailed me, sent cards, and most importantly, prayed for Elise. Thank you, thank you, thank you. Please continue to pray for her.

I am terrified of my cervix. I don't want it to shorten one more millimeter. I am in bed every second of every day with my feet raised above my head; I'm sort of on an incline to keep as much pressure off the cervix as possible. It is 10 steps from the bed to the loo, and I am afraid to take them. I don't go to the bathroom until it's evident that I'm either to take those 10 steps or wet the bed. And there is no terror like the strain of a bowel movement, so you can just imagine what point I allow myself to reach before taking my 10-step journey. If going to the bathroom is a life or death issue for me, then imagine getting in a car and taking a nice bumpy, hour-long trip to the doctor's office.

The Dreaded Appointment

We arrived at the medical offices and got a "Front Row Joe" (primo parking space). This was good news to someone who is afraid to take 10 steps to visit the loo. My husband opened the door and went into the lobby to let them know I was coming and would need to lie down and not wait in the waiting room. While I waited in the car I saw a healthy preggo walking up to the door where she was surprised to be met by a friend who asked her how pregnant she was. "38 weeks," came the reply. They both entered the door pleasantly gabbing away.

My husband returned and got me out of the car. The first office door opens into a small foyer with two doors. One door leads to the OB offices while the other leads to GYN. "Li'l Miss 38 Weeks" was *still* standing there in the cramped foyer gabbing her head off with her hand on the door handle while I was praying that Elise wouldn't fall out on the floor during the gab fest. It reminds me of those absolutely oblivious folks who stop, one in each lane, to have a nice little chat in the middle of the road as people racing to funerals and emergency rooms wait fuming behind them.

"Excuse me." I said pointedly.

"Blah, blah, blah," said the motor mouth to her friend. "Blah, blah, blah and gab, gab, gab." Translation: "I am oblivious."

I sighed heavily and went to open the door that she still clung to. I rolled my eyes at her as my husband said, "My wife needs to enter the building."

Gabby Pants, finally realizing that she shared the world with other people, released her grip on the door and got out of the way. I shot all the way through to the exam room, which my doctor entered chuckling to see me lying upside down on the exam table in order to maintain my heels-over-head Trendelenburg position.

"You don't have to stand on your head this whole pregnancy," Dr. Keanu said.

"I will," I informed.

"Don't I know it," said he who knows it.

He looked at the perinatologist's diagnosis/opinion from last Friday and said, "OK, let's do the cerclage."

"Whoa, whoa, whoa!" said my husband and I, "Let's talk about this!"

Dr. Keanu indulged.

We tried to explore the subject in order to determine whether the benefit of cerclage outweighed the risks at this point. The thing with an incompetent cervix is: it's a gamble. Especially with my particular measurements. The bottom line was that we didn't know. We didn't know if we could get by without the cerclage, and we didn't know if she would live one more day after the cerclage was placed. If she makes it four more weeks she will have a chance, a *chance*. Fifty percent. Better odds than today's. Today she will die if born. One hundred percent probability. **She will die.**

Dr. Keanu really listened to our concerns. I knew it had already been a long day for him. I tried to personalize the issue.

"Pretend," I said, "that when Elise grows up she will be the one to find the cure for cancer, AIDS, Parkinson's and any other disease you can think of. Pretend that she will find the cure and develop it into one pill, one pill that costs $2. If this were really so, can you imagine how important she would be to the world? Well, that's how important she is to us already."

Dr. Keanu knows that I get HG, and he knows how bad it is. He is aware that this is our last pregnancy, win or lose. It seems to mean something to him, and for that we are glad. But it's kind of silly when you think about it: Children are not expendable one way or the other. If it is your last pregnancy or if you intend to have 10 more, each time it's your only shot at *that* child and that child's only shot at his or her life. It's *always* the "last chance" if you think in realistic terms; it's *always* so very important.

They measured my cervix again: no change in two days. They pressed on the uterus as though they were trying to squish Elise out, and my cervix shortened a millimeter. Thanks loads. No funneling, just shortening. Shortening increases my risk of preterm labor as we all know and fear.

I asked Dr. Keanu a slew of questions through streaming tears. He confided that if it were he and his wife he didn't know what they would do either. He said that my history with carrying my son to term was good. He said that the contractions that I am having are not. He said that not funneling and not dilating so far is good. He said that losing six millimeters in 14 days of bed rest is not. He said the cerclage could kill her. He said not getting the cerclage could kill her. He said opting for either would be reasonable at this point and what, oh what did we want to do?

Go time. Time for the answer to a life or death question. No pressure here.

"I can't give you an answer," I said. "I'm not going to do the cerclage today, I'll tell you that much. I might not do it at all."

He was not shocked. He was not opinionated, oppositional or cruel. In fact, it seemed rather reasonable to him. Hubby felt the same way. No cerclage. He wasn't comfortable with it. We sort of decided to shift the paradigm a little. We could not get an answer as to whether bed rest or cerclage would give Elise the best chance, so we began looking at it as if she were going to die. If she were going to die, which could we live with: She died because we did something that killed her or she died because we didn't do something that might have saved her? Selfish, but we've so little to go on.

Bed rest is not "doing nothing." For anyone who has ever been on bed rest for months, you know it is SOMETHING. The moments I most look forward to in the day are the moments when I am forced to take my 10 steps to the loo. I'm terrified, but I am sitting up, and my body is so thankful then. The weight is off my back, the painful pockets of trapped air release themselves in a hail of burps and other less pleasant emissions. I can breathe, my blood flows out of my head. All of this relief lasts a glorious 45 seconds. And then the crucial moment comes: the TP exam. If there is blood I will fly to the doctor's screaming for a cerclage. If there is none I will thank God and take five steps back to the foot of my elevated bed where I will slither my body back into position.

Supine dining is no picnic. In fact my appetite has decreased significantly. The moment I swallow, gravity is not working to my benefit. I feel that everything is lodged just in my esophagus. And the toast and cracker crumbs make me feel as though I'm receiving constant, crumby "acupressure therapy." It is like having a sunburned back and sleeping in a bed full of sand and crushed sea shells. Bed rest is *not* nothing. This is an alternative to cerclage, and for the time being we have chosen it.

Yesterday I felt more peaceful about it than I do today. About an hour ago I had one contraction that was particularly nasty. My uterus became hard as a rock. These are not Braxton Hicks. Dr. Keanu says those don't happen until later in the pregnancy. These are abnormal and troubling contractions. But not so troubling that he did anything about them other than to warn of their unusual quality. It's just one more thing on the plate.

I'm full, thanks. May I be excused?

We hope we made the right decision. It worked with our son, although we do realize this is a different pregnancy, and things have definitely not followed suit.

Please keep praying. Specifically, pray for Elise's survival, for the cervix to stay closed with no funneling, for miraculous LENGTHENING, and also pray for the contractions to stop. *Please.*

I am 20 weeks and working on my second day. With each passing day we get closer to the dream of a long life with Elise. Each day is a step away from profound grief and a step toward wordless rapture. I can't help feeling though that I am twisting in the wind. I want some sort of oracle, some sort of soothsaying vane to direct my attention to the way this all will end. I feel helpless to save my vulnerable little girl. I desperately want God to intervene and prevent her death. I want the pink, happy ribbon on my hospital door 20 short weeks from now. I do *not* want, affixed to my door, the dark picture of the weeping leaf.

This is the valley of the shadow, and I have no option but to walk through it. It is scary, it is sad. But I am not alone.

Saturday, January 10, 2004

Still hanging in there. I am *so sore* from bed rest. I need to get those "thigh calluses" again so it doesn't feel like my hip bones are coming through my skin. It wakes me up all night. My aching hips say, "Turn, for goodness' sake, turn!" And just when it seems I've only been on the right side for five minutes I am waking up again with an urgency to turn on my left. ARGH! Later I will see a commercial with a little girl dressed in a frilly, pink dress, and nothing will matter but getting Elise to term.

By the way, I have neglected to mention that everything always smells like cigarettes and no one smokes. This pregnancy is insane! And only 19 more weeks, folks!

Yes, yes! Only 19 more weeks of my whining! If all goes well that is.

Also, I was paired up with a great support on the Sidelines Web site. She also had HG and IC and chose bed rest instead of cerclage. She had funneling and only half a centimeter left to her cervix! She also delivered her daughter on her due date! And her little one was over *11 pounds*! I have talked to my support on the phone, and although I am still scared out of my mind, I feel much more hopeful and calm. It's a beautiful thing! This doesn't mean I've gone lax with my bed rest.

I have gotten a bedside potty to further express my commitment. And the best part ever is that my husband has to clean it! **MUHAHAHAHAAAAAAAA!!!**

While he loudly protests the grotesque nature of his job I lie here and snicker. He cleans the removable bucket, fills it with ice, and I pee like a highlander for the rest of the day. For the bucket we abide by Creole plumbing laws: "If it's pee let it be; If it's brown flush it down." But when I consider what I've been through and what he's been through in comparison, I think about breaking that law! And when he comes in here messin' with me about bacon, something that just sends nauseous shivers up and down my spine, I *seriously* want to bless him with some bedside potty Tootsie Rolls!

It's OK, though. I had a truckload of asparagus last night, and his gagged retching was music to my ears! Can you say "toxic paper mill wasteland?" Hey, I'm on bed rest 24/7; I get my kicks where I can.

P.S.
All my hair is falling out, so in addition to being fatter and more uncomfortable the next time I write, I will also be bald. If fortunes in cookies were real my husband would have been warned.

Tuesday, January 13, 2004

Went to the doctor's today. Good news! There is no funneling, no dilation, and cervix has not shortened. In fact, it has lengthened! It is now 2.6 or 2.7 cm (out of 4 cm)! Good deal! Lengthen and strengthen! Keep praying!

Elise kicks her hello to you as I type this!

Three more weeks and we reach the stage of "viability" whatever *that* is. Babies have been born at 21 weeks and survived. "Viability" has more to do with technology than the baby's livability. Why, in 100 years they might be able to keep a 12-weeker alive. At any rate, I turned 21 weeks yesterday. I hope and pray we make it for at least three more weeks.

Doc said I can get off bed rest at eight months or so if I make it that far. I hope to! I'd get out of bed right around my birthday. That'd be a grand gift!

Potty Talk

Because I have issues with my cervix I don't really want to be sitting on the pot straining for poo to put it bluntly. I don't know if that has any effect on the cervix, but it can't be good. So one of my missions in life right now is to make my dookie endeavors as easy-breezy as possible. This involves the daily consumption of such things as bran, fruit, veggies and prune juice. So far so good. However, these foodstuffs do pose a problem for this Jumpin' Jack Ash: it's a gas, gas, gas. (I'm such a nerd.)

The doc was a good sport and began telling me about the benefits of a good dose of simethicone when he was interrupted by my husband who had a better, drug-free solution. The doc and I yielded the floor while we listened in earnest for the alternative. All eyes on him, my husband grabbed my finger and began yanking on it saying, "This is the 'pull-my-finger' method, and it always works for me!" I made a few fart noises and we all had a good laugh.

The doc left the room and gave us a minute to gather ourselves before the sonogram tech was to come back in to help me off the table. As soon as the door closed a nice gas bubble settled right down to the bottom of things and, believing we had a few moments, I let it rip. It was silent but oh-so-deadly. My husband giggled at his newly singed eyebrows, and I remarked that the tech had better not come in for a while if she knew what was good for her. No sooner had the words left my mouth when the unfortunate tech stepped unaware into an atomic mushroom cloud.

"Do you think she smelled it?" my husband later asked in genuine wonder. I looked at him incredulously and replied, "People in New Zealand smelled it!"

So our visit was wonderful and really stank! Thank God you weren't there! (No, really!)

Thursday, January 15, 2004

Hello, all. Elise has started hiccupping. I could feel it for the first time the day before yesterday. For those who wonder what that's like, it's a steady, rhythmic pulsing. It's adorable and very human. Roe v. Wade says Elise is not a human but a mass of tissue. A mass of hiccupping tissue. They know better. We all do. Even Roe herself now opposes abortion. But it's still happening. Right now someone Elise's age is being aborted. My God, what are we doing?

Elise was very quiet yesterday. It was one of those slow days. After not feeling any movement for three or so hours, I sort of started to worry. The moment my son came home from school and said, "Hi, Mom," Tummy Lumpkin did a somersault.

"Oh boy, my big brother's home!"

There is a five-year difference between them, but I hope they will be close. Maybe it will be easier for them because they will be homeschooled.

Again with the Potty Talk

Sorry to broach this subject again; I know you all are getting sick of it. But I have to tell you that my husband forgot to dump the bedside yesterday morning before going to work. To keep it short and relatively sweet let me just say P.U. It was cosmic justice for the asparagus episode the other day. Waves of yellow stench wafted around the room and I became desperate. The prospect of lying here in this room all day with *that* was pretty unthinkable. I tried to think of someone I could call for such a dastardly job. Funny thing is, I thought of at least six people

I could ask. There's a saying that if you can count five true friends then you're lucky. Lucky is one thing, but you know you are *blessed* when you can count more than five people who would come into your smelly room and dump out a stinky bucket of all-night pee. Thank you, God, for the pee dumpers in my life!

I won't say the name of the person who came yesterday to relieve me (no pun intended), but she's a bright girl, and I told her I'd give her props in today's entry. So here you go, friend! Your efforts literally went to waste, and I thank you very much for that! You can count on me to dump your stinky pee pot if ever urine need.

Snicker.

Tuesday, January 20, 2004

I haven't written for a few days. Not because anything is the matter but simply to avoid clone posts about bedside potties and related activities. Nothing much happens when you are in bed 24 hours a day.

For this diary the rule is:

No news is good news.

We are still hanging in there. Elise had a couple of slow days and then a day or so of nearly kicking my guts out. It's encouraging. Each movement cheers me on. "Hang in there, Mama."

Emotionally, I have caught myself wanting to cry a few times. I'm frustrated because my eating is dwindling even more. I'm not gaining enough weight and will probably start losing weight soon at this rate. It's all this tilted lying down. I want to get up and play with my son, get my life back, yadda, yadda, yadda. So I get frustrated, and my eyes start to well up with tears that I have no business spilling. I think back to those inhuman times in the midst of severe HG. I get sick to my stomach just recalling it. I sweat as my mind fogs over; it does not want to remember such a thing. Those days were songless. Suffering, like a cancer, consumed every aspect of my being. I couldn't even afford to be interested in anything other than getting through each moment. I hung on by a fingernail. I would rather die than know that suffering again.

Presently I have knocked over a gigantic glass of strawberry milk. It is soaking into the carpet as I type. I can't do anything about it except sign off and place a phone call to someone who will come and clean it up. If no one answers I'm going to have one sour mess in here. It serves me right for drinking strawberry milk in the first place. Who *does* that!

This Just In

Just got an email from another HG mom who is pregnant and feels that she wants to either kill herself or end the pregnancy to make the vomiting stop. I can understand completely, and if you've been reading this diary from the start, perhaps you can understand a little bit too. Please pray for her. She is in agony and has a long way to go.

Monday, January 26, 2004

This is one of the crucial weeks. Week 24. Day one. This is the ever elusive "viability week." "Viability" is a term often so creatively defined that it has virtually lost all meaning. Yet my pregnancy book says this is the viability week. If we can make it through this week, Elise will have a chance of surviving. She would most likely have severe handicaps (i.e., special needs for the politically correct set) but she's got a shot at life! 44% by some accounts.

So pray us through this week and more, people. Pray because I have been feeling "funny," and that is never good. For the E.R. watchers who can handle graphic descriptions:

A big blob of mucus on the tissue yesterday and "loose" stool today. Let's hope it's a fluke. A big yucky fluke.

She has been sleeping pretty much all morning. Last night she squirmed so that I started getting motion sickness from her movement! Her daddy comes in and talks to her sometimes and she will stop whatever she is doing to listen. It is funny. She literally stops with his voice and starts moving again when he's quiet. This one is a daddy's girl for sure.

Lots and lots of hiccups.

I enjoy the rest when she is still, but I worry. I don't want her to be *still*-still! So now of course I'm thinking she's dead because it has been an hour. Ow! A nice little reminder that all is well. Ahhhh...

I have never known the luxury of a confident pregnancy. And I never will. That's a bit upsetting. Alas.

Big Punkin Butt came in here last night and crawled under the covers that the "baw head dog" (hairless cat) had been under for hours. Big PB stuck his head out and said "PU! It smells like Kitty's underpitts in here!" Now I'm thinking of marketing kitty roll-on. Just kidding. My kid makes me laugh—what can I say?

OK, boring entry. I told you it was going to get like this. That's why I don't often post.

I go to the doctor's tomorrow. I should be getting steroid injections in the near future. These will hopefully improve Elise's chances, because they stimulate lung function, and that is a biggie in preemies.

Well, I've got to go and watch back-to-back episodes of A Baby Story on TLC, so the moms can all talk about how surprisingly wonderful pregnancy is, and I can cry when they pop their little blue babies out. I always bawl when I see a baby being born. I'm a sucker. Maybe I'll see you tomorrow. Same time, same channel.

Tuesday, January 27, 2004

Got back from the doc's not too long ago. I have gained approximately 4 more millimeters on the cervix! I now have a solidly normal measurement! This doesn't mean I have a normal cervix. If I get up and start moving around some it will go back down. Dr. Keanu said, "Looks like bed rest and prayer are working!" Amen!

He says he'll probably do the steroid injections at 26 weeks. Sounds reasonable. My hospital uses the stupid kind of steroids that are inconvenient. For two days I have to travel to the big city every 12 hours to get injections. It's dexamethasone. Betamethasone only requires two shots, one every 24 hours. That would be better, as we have to travel quite a way to get to the office. The car makes me queasy. I asked if I could just shoot myself up at home. He said no because they are "IM." What the heck does that mean? I had to remind him I wasn't a doctor. I think sometimes he forgets. D'har.

IM means intramuscular as opposed to subcutaneous. I've only been giving myself subcues in this pregnancy. IMs have to go deeper. I was surprised that I wasn't allowed to impale myself at home. With all the other stuff they expected us to do during home health care I figured they'd just ask me to check in after I delivered my own baby. It seems we can manage tubes just outside our hearts but we can't stab ourselves in the butt. Alrighty.

I was surprised to learn that I gained 5 pounds. I'll have to send Pepperidge Farm a thank you note.

We got to see Tummy Lumpkin pretty well today. Her spine and ribs are so intricate and fascinating. A person within a person; I'm a walking miracle.

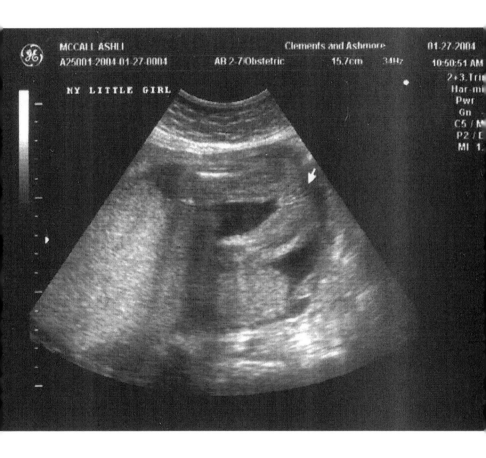

She's still a girl. She stuck her little butt right up to the transducer. I guess she wanted us to know what she thought about all that. Her little cookie is so obviously a little cookie. Can cookies be cute? Hers is! We took a picture.

I spat on the doctor. It was an accident. I was trying to say the word "swollen" with a German accent, and the spit in the middle of my teeth went flying across the room like a fluffy white UFO. He saw it. We all saw it. I should have said, "Whoa, did someone turn on a sprinkler in here?" or "Hey I should just say it, not spray it!" but instead I just turned red and kept on talking. It can be embarrassing or funny. Today I chose embarrassing.

When I spat on him I was trying to tell him how swollen my face looked. I.e., "My faze is all svollen!" In an attempt at reassuring me he said, "I think it looks fine. It was much fatter last time I saw you." Uhhh…

We talked about cramping and gas and poop, and my husband pinched his nose and pointed at me. Dr. Keanu ignored him while I giggled uncontrollably.

Dr. visits are always a hoot when you get good news.

Keep praying for Elise.

Doctor's orders.

Friday, January 30, 2004

Today is black Friday, the 7th anniversary of my first child's death. I almost didn't remember it. I woke up and it seemed like any other day. The only thing amiss was feeling oddly concerned for my son's safety. I kept hoping nothing would happen that would take his life. Images of car wrecks or crazed schoolyard shooters flickered through my mind. Why? I couldn't grasp it. Was it a warning?

No. It was a memory.

Someone I loved, a child of mine, died a very gruesome, violent death seven years ago. It is in there, in my heart and mind, even when I forget to remember.

I am thinking of who that child must have been and what s/he must have looked like, sounded like, smelled like—the whole package. I wish I could remember my life without this stone. I forget who I was; I only know me without Tennessee.

I struggled to get through that pregnancy, but other than that, I never got to love my child. I gave up. I cried Uncle. I never got to love Tennessee.

For Tennessee

I'm not allowed to love you.

The "pro-life" movement says

I can only feel forgiven and set free.

The "pro-choice" movement says

I can only feel liberated and grateful.

Death says

feelings are moot.

Gears spin

as abortion snaps a belt

in the machine of adoration.

Vats of earmarked love

grease broken apparatuses,

fueling the unhappiness

of life without you

and days that remember

your black passing,

reverberating forever

in the vacuum of time.

February

Monday, February 02, 2004

It's 3:30 A.M. I've been up since two with a stuffed nose and sore throat courtesy of my five-year-old. I'm thinking strep. I'll make hubby miss work to take me for a culture.

I love Elise. I really, really love Elise, but my body will be eternally grateful when this pregnancy is over. Some women are well-oiled baby-making machines, and some women (like me) were not built for that action. In a bygone world I would have already died in pregnancy. I'm not naturally meant to have children, but I snuck and did it anyway.

Boy, I just did not need this little ailment on top of everything else. Eating has gotten so hard again. I guess it's being sick that's doing it. Can't wait for more fever blisters. I always get them after any kind of infection.

What am I going to do for the rest of the morning? I am not tired, and I am sick of the Internet and TV. I have been reading this book called *Lime Five*, but I don't feel like picking that up right now. When I'm a well person I can only read small portions of it; it's way too heavy for sick reading. I know, I know, you're thinking: "*How* can you be reading a book like *that* when you're pregnant?!" Everyone ought to read it when they're pregnant. Maybe they'd be more sympathetic to the plight of those involved. As it is everyone thinks we sick preggies are the very ones for whom abortion was invented. Well guess what. That's not good enough. We don't *want* abortion, **we want help.** Please don't give up on us.

Elise has been jogging on her treadmill. It seems like she has finally settled in for a nap. A little girl—wow! What's that all about? I can't wait!

It's 8:30 A.M.

I have vomited a couple of times and have lots of diarrhea. I started having panic attacks right around the time I started vomiting. I don't get panic attacks in normal life. They're really hard for me to understand. I can't deny that they exist, because I'm having them. My husband says it's because the vomiting is triggering feelings that relate to the HG. I don't know what it is, but I hate it. It's such a bad feeling. I know that the vomiting and constant trips to the real toilet (a luxury) are putting pressure on the cervix. I can feel it. So I realize I am worried for Elise. But I've been so worried for her before and not had panic attacks. How is this all going to end?

Today is the first day of my 25th week. In other words, I'm only 24 weeks. It's the point of "viability," and that is a good thing, however I have a friend whose baby was born at 25 weeks three months ago, and he is still in the neonatal intensive care unit (NICU) with severe lung disease and lots of other problems. It's not that I fear the burden of a disabled child, I just don't want Elise to have to go through all of that. Also, even though 24 weeks is the point of "viability," the odds aren't fantastic. She could still die. The point is, she does *not* need to be born right now, and all of this puking and diarrhea is not helping her and is freaking me out.

Oh dear God, please help me.

Please pray for us. Please!

Thursday, February 05, 2004

I'm feeling somewhat better. I'm still sick but no throwing up and no more Hershey squirts. Man, I haven't said "Hershey squirts" since high school. Perhaps there's a reason why.

Anyway, I ate dinner last night. It was the first meal I've had since getting sick. It's still hard to eat, so I try to watch TV during meals; it helps me to ignore the food.

I eat at around 7 P.M. when That '70s Show comes on. Not the best viewing choice, but it takes my mind off of serious things. "Eric's" real name is Topher, which is the coolest name in history. It's like his parents couldn't decide whether to name him Tofu or Gopher. You have to love it.

I thought, for a millisecond, about naming my daughter Dixie or Cricket, but I couldn't decide between the two, and "Dicket" didn't sound too cool.

Friday, February 06, 2004

I don't know what is going on with me, because I am just getting better with this cold/flu thing, yet still I had another bizarre "panic attack" last night. My heart was beating a million miles a minute and I couldn't tell if that was causing the weird anxiety or if the weird anxiety was causing the racing heartbeat. Whatever it is, it SUCKS. It can have a tendency to happen right when I'm falling asleep. Does anyone know of any medical condition that would cause such symptoms? Or is it sheer lunacy?

I am currently getting kicked in the cervix. Do you even *know* what this feels like? Stay away from the trap door, Baby!

It is storming here. I have been obsessively watching TV to determine what Friday's weather will be. If it is as bad as this I don't let my little boy go over to his grandparents, because I just know they will get into a car accident and die on the way there. Gee, my behavior isn't weird is it? I don't take chances anymore. I have learned that yes, it can happen to me—and usually does!

A pal called last night and said she delivered her baby in her midwife's new Durango on the way to the birthing center. She is one of these extraordinary people who can have natural pregnancies and births. She actually has the option of the hippie home birth and has done it a gazillion times. Freaks like me are required to be hooked up to meds and things in a hospital setting during birth in case anything goes wrong at the culmination of a high risk pregnancy.

My hippy pal said she had labored for hours and the baby just wasn't coming out. Finally, she asked to be taken to the hospital for drugs and a c-section. If you knew this uber hippy woman your eyes would have just popped out and rolled around on the floor. She explained, "Well, I was suffering too much not to see any results after several hours. I just wanted them to cut that baby out of me!"

Cut the baby out?

I told her I knew how she felt.

Her midwife implored her to go to the birth center and try, so she got out of the kiddie pool in her living room and got into the midwife's new Durango. Two miles down the road the baby's head popped out. Oopsie! The value on the Durango immediately dropped. They pulled over and the midwife finished the job.

Congrats, Mama and Baby Durango!

I know a couple more people who get to have their babies in the next few months. And then it's *my* turn!

Saturday, February 07, 2004

Still hanging in there. No bizarre-o panic attacks in 24 hours. This is good. I am almost 25 weeks! Of course my goal is always to make it through the next hour, but my *big* next goal is 28 weeks. We make it to 28 weeks, and it's Welch's sparkling grape juice, baby! Speaking of which, I got some this year for New Year's and it had a TWIST OFF CAP! What the *heck* is *that* all about? I always remembered it having a plastic pop-off cork. It's not mock champagne if you have to twist off the cap. Might as well drink it out of a paper sack.

Bath day today! I always know when it's bath day because the buzzards start circling.

Anyhoo, I'm going to go watch cartoons with Li'l Buddy. Spongebob is on. Hmmm, I wonder if Courage the Cowardly Dog is on today. Rats! I think I've already missed Mystery Science Theatre 3000! I need a TV guide. Television has become my life. Pathetic.

Monday, February 09, 2004

I am 25 weeks. This is officially the first day of the 26th week! I go to Dr. Keanu on Thursday, and I will have the option of beginning corticosteroids at that time. Four shots over a 24-hour period. Should I do it? Feel free to weigh in on the decision. Do you know something that I don't? Tell me!

Eating is getting better! To illustrate this I ate half a bag of Baken-ets hot and spicy pork rinds last night and am salivating now as I look at the half-full bag. I may see the *glass* half-empty, but a bag of pork rinds is always half full. Mmm, pork rinds!

Look at them just sitting there mocking me. They *know* I can't eat them until noon. That's my rule. If I wait until noon I can convince myself that I'm not really an addict and that I can control it and quit anytime I want to.

FYI, the proper southern pronunciation for "pork rinds" is "poke rhines."

Baken-ets. I mention the brand name, because there is no other pork rind worthy of being eaten. Oh, I have sampled many a rind, my friends, but Baken-ets is far superior to any other, and I'm willing to fist-fight anyone who doesn't think so!

You know…I could just have *one* now and then the rest at noon. ARG! No! Even though I *could*, I mustn't! I am master of the pork rind, not the other way around. The Bible says I must not let the pork rind make me its slave. (Somewhere in I Corinthians. Chapter six, I think.) I must resist the pork rind! Only 40 more minutes and then it's hog heaven. Mmmmm!

What will I do until then? Oh! I know! I'll eat some peanut butter cookies. Coooookies! Peanut butter cookies and pork rinds. Elvis would be proud.

Tuesday, February 10, 2004

Let's talk about disappointment, shall we? First, I would like all to know that yes, I *did* wait until noon, only just, to dine on the "rine," oh yes, I did. And after such a delightful appetizer I opened my Spongebob Squarepants sandwich keeper salivating for what I knew would be a delicious Boar's Head ham and dill havarti sammich on pumpernickel/sourdough swirl bread. Much to my utter dismay, staring back at me was a Boar's Head ham and dill havarti cheese sammy on CINNAMON RAISIN swirl bread.

Let me say it again:

ham, cheese, mustard, and mayo on sweet cinnamon/raisin bread.

Mustard and dill on cinnamon toast with raisins.

Any takers?

Men.

I called my husband to berate him. That's right, the guy can't catch a break for trying. But seriously, *really*, what was he thinking? He was sorry, so, so sorry, but I was now without lunch! Sorry will not produce a sammy on the proper bread! "Eat your yogurt," he advised. "Fine," I said succinctly and hung up.

I slid the yogurt out of the cooler and read the label: Strawberry yogurt. A printed banner around the tub said something like: "Now with room for mixing in your own fun flavors!" In other words, the 8-ounce cup now only contains 6 ounces of yogurt. Less yogurt, same price. How novel. Ah well. I opened the top and then reached for my spoon. My spoon. Where is my spoon?

"Where is my spoon?" I asked my husband in yet another phone call to his office. "D'oh!" he replied.

He asked me to help him remember such things. I asked him if he needed me to remind him to wipe his butt after a good healthy poop, a healthy poop that I myself would not be having since I had no lunch!

Yes, everyone wants to be married to me.

Wednesday, February 11, 2004

Nothing to tell today. Just another day. I guess I'll rattle a little bit so you don't forget about me.

Elise

The little girl is doing well. She tumbles around making womb mischief all the live-long day. She got the hiccups seven different times on Monday. Somewhere before the hundredth hiccup she decided she had had enough. She tried to kick them away. Already a no-nonsense girl.

I have started back on milk products just three days ago. This was a first after the lovely puke/squirt flu. I've been trying to drink strawberry milk, and my stomach just rolls. I wonder what impression this makes on a little girl who can hear every gurgle. Monsters in the closet? She doesn't know the half of it.

The last couple to be due before me just had their baby. It's my turn next. I've got such a long way to go.

Nine and one-half weeks until I can get out of bed and I am counting the days. Who am I kidding? I am counting the MOMENTS!

When I got preggo we bought a new bed. It's an adjustable bed kind of like a hospital bed. I got it in a king and spent over $2,000 thinking it would serve me well during the pregnancy and then just be a luxury afterwards. Now I hate this confounded bed so much! This is the sick bed. I have lived and died in this damnable contraption and all I want is out! This is my prison! I want to burn it!

Ugh, I am, as usual, sick to my stomach. On the verge of puking but never quite there anymore. And of course, Elise has the hiccups.

Thursday, February 12, 2004

Saw Dr. Keanu today and the cervix measured in at 3.4 cm! Dr. Keanu said, "Sheesh, how long can a human cervix get?" He said that what is happening to the measurement is "unusual." Hey, you can't put God in a box. Keep praying, people!

:-)

I start steroid injections tomorrow night. This is going to be a pain in the butt. Literally. We drive 30 minutes to the hospital to get the shot at 10 and have to be there by 10 the next morning for another shot. Then we have to be there at 10 at night for another shot and again for another shot at 10 on Sunday morning. Shots, shots, shots. You wish you could have them, but they are all mine! 2bad4U.

Dr. Keanu said that in addition to maturing Elise's lungs, the shots may also help me eat a little better for a few days.

Going to be up a lot with all these shots. And a glucose test soon. And another Dr.'s appointment in two weeks plus another doctor's appointment three days later for the 4D sonogram. The nurse tried to get me to schedule it for later because she said I'd get better pictures. I told her I wanted it at 28 weeks and she just shook her head.

Everyone (except Dr. Keanu) was really grumpy today at the office. I actually got into a nice little argument with one of the nurses. They are all so disgusted by my huffing and puffing when I walk, because they have no clue what it's like to be on strict bed rest. I lost lots of muscle tone and energy. I take a bath, and I'm so tired I have to sleep for the following 10 hours. They don't get it. They think I'm just trying to get attention. If

I wanted to get attention, I would do it in such a way as to elicit *positive* attention, hello. What I'd like more than anything would be to get *no* attention. I'd like to be a normal, average preggo, but I don't get to. Ever. So let's all just deal with it, shall we? I hate to tell them, but the huffing and puffing is just going to get worse as time goes on. I guess they can just sit and stew with their crummy, negative, incorrect assumptions. What a blessing their attitudes will be to them and their sick patients. Bleah. Negativity is contagious.

I ate French fries and a hamburger on the way home. A hamburger with onions no less. Raw onions! I have a feeling I'm going to pay.

Tuesday, February 17, 2004

I am a huge, huge cow. Elise weighs around 2 pounds, but you would think I was 20 months pregnant. With 14 more weeks to go I simply cannot fathom how I could possibly get any bigger. I am massive. My face is fat, my body is completely distorted, and I am absolutely gorgeous! I am never so beautiful as when I am carrying a tiny li'l tummy traveler. I cannot believe I have made it this far.

This is the second day of my 27th week. I.e., I'm only 26 weeks. Ugh. Next week will begin the third trimester for us, the last third of a Technicolor nightmare. The days stretch themselves out before me; I can hardly stand it. I love my daughter, I love the way I look with her body in mine, but my God in Heaven, this can't be over soon enough.

Monday, yesterday, lasted two weeks. How could it be such a long day? How can I complain now? I've been in worse places physically. Vomiting every eight minutes for an entire day—that was a bad, long day. Lying in a bed for the 21st week, just lying here, not puking or soiling myself and even having the ability to eat—well, I should feel home free. But I don't. I want out of this confounded bed.

I feel sorry for myself and then remember why I am in this bed. I am in this bed because I aborted my first child in the second trimester, due to HG and the lack of good medical support, and this permanently damaged my cervix. Two of us walked into that building, but only one of us walked out. I was the lucky one.

My child lost his/her life and I got off with a booboo on my cervix. I saw the jar they stuffed him/her in, yet here I am feeling sorry for myself. I am in this bed with my guts rolling back into my throat and my digestive system unable to function properly. Whatever your position on the issue, this is the consequence of aborting my baby seven years ago. I made the bed I'm in.

Nine more weeks and then I can get up. That's all I want now. Just to get up, walk around, clean the house, do the dishes, cook dinner and be my son's mommy. Nine weeks. Over 60 days. 60 days?! *60 more days like this?!?* Sigh...

It could be worse. Obviously.

Wednesday, February 18, 2004

Poopy-doopy is very active lately. Squirmin' roun', squirmin' roun'. It's so great to feel her, but she makes me seasick! Her brother is sick, sick, sick. Diarrhea and not much eating. My husband's hands are cracked and bleeding from washing his hands so often. He's being so careful trying not to spread this stuff to me. Oh honeychile, that's all I need.

I'm going to write a song for you now because I am bored.

Ode to Heartburn and Gas

Heartburn and gas,
heartburn and gas.
Lawsy, lawsy!
Heartburn and gas!

Give me some meds:
cherry flavored pills,
a bottle of Tums
to cure all my ills.
Oh lawsy!
Lawsy, lawsy!
Heartburn and gas!

I shunna et that Reuben on rye:
corned beef and sour kraut—
I'm a'gonna die!
I'm not gonna make it!
I'm not gonna last
because of this heartburn,
this heartburn and gas!

Oh lawsy!
Lawsy, lawsy!
Heartburn and gas,
heartburn and gas!

Feel me, feel my pain;
take me a bath
and wash it down the drain!
Give me more fiber
so I don't have to strain!
Make it so easy

for me to pass
& get through this heartburn,
this heartburn and gas!

Lawsy!
Lawsy, oh lawsy!
Heartburn,
heartburn and gas!

Someone set that to music. Feel free to add a nice flatulent denouement, package it up, and send it to me. I'll give you a cookie, but you won't want to eat it, because I'll touch it for sure, without washing my hands.

Thursday, February 19, 2004

I was having coffee with God this morning when I read something simple yet profound regarding John 2:10, Jesus' first miracle:

"God always saves the best wine until last, but Satan starts with his best and then leads the sinner into suffering and perhaps even death."

I have found this to be so true, particularly in this pregnancy. The worst was first. I had horrible times to go through. I could reject those times and curse everyone around me or I could submit to those times and be a blessing. I could learn nothing and live in deeper sorrow or I could suffer like a dog for a while and then gain character, understanding, perspective, fullness, love, a deeper, more real relationship with God, etc.

Evil says, "Here, here is your solution! The best thing for you right here, right now at this moment! Come, take advantage of this beautiful cure! Why should you suffer? Why should anyone suffer? You can be free! Why wait? Freedom now!"

But oh the deception! The sheen on that apple is poison.

God will allow you to suffer, to work your butt off to survive. It will prove you, it will build character in you, it will be anything but easy. But it is for your own good and the good of those around you if you submit and find the sense in your terrible suffering. If you refuse and resist, if you choose the best evil has to offer, you damn yourself to abominable consequences.

It seems so glaringly obvious. It's a quiet, simple truth. It is pure and real and something to hang onto in a lost world full of so much suffering.

Whatever we see, whatever hell we go through, press on. Get your hands dirty, cover them with blisters of faith! God is saving the best for last. Count on it!

Friday, February 20, 2004

57 more days in bed. I am trying to tell myself that 57 days aren't much. "I can do this," I half-lie. Ugh. 57 days. I think I'd be dealing with it a little better if I felt totally healthy.

I still suffer from constant nausea. Yesterday I almost threw up. I got to the toilet and knew it was coming. "Oh please, please, don't let me puke, God!" My stomach rolled. Gurgle, gurgle. But I didn't throw up. At the last second it stifled itself. That is the closest I've come to throwing up from pregnancy nausea since the hospital. I have to eat constantly or I get sick. By dinner I am just *ill*. Sometimes I think I'll never be able to get it down, but down it somehow goes and then things get a little better. Is this how it is for normal pregnant ladies in that hackneyed "first trimester?" Is this what "morning sickness" is? I wouldn't know. I've never had it. Ugh. Gripe, gripe, gripe.

In addition to being in bed, being sore from being in bed, having bad digestion from being in bed, being nauseous (exacerbated by being in bed), I have had the nastiest taste in my mouth since the dawn of this pregnancy. It tastes like caustic metal. Caustic, mediciney metal. Yum. Will it ever go away? It's not what caused my ptyalism (inability to swallow spit without throwing up and needing to constantly spit in a cup), but it didn't help, and it still sucks eggs.

Ptyalism. Ugh. It got so bad that I had to sleep with a washcloth in my mouth. At one point I had a tube in each arm, a tube in my leg, a vomit basin by my head and a washcloth in my mouth soaking with viscid saliva all night long. That's how I slept! With alarms going off three times a night. BEEP! BEEP! My bag is empty! I need a new bag! Back to sleep for an hour. BEEP! BEEP! My Zofran is empty! I need a new syringe! Back to sleep for an hour. BEEP! BEEP! My CADD pump battery is dying! I need a new battery! Help, God, HELP! Barf, barf! I am literally getting teary-eyed remembering it. How did I ever get through that? How? It is a miracle. I was there: I know.

Am I going to need serious therapy to deal with having been through this illness this time? It is not as upsetting as "not" getting through a hyperemetic pregnancy, but this little pink passenger has taken me on a different trip! A long, lingering, traumatic trip. It really kind of freaks me out to look back at where I've been. I'm surprised, because in spite of the fact that no one died I'm still incredibly shell-shocked. What a fight! I am so tired of fighting.

When this is over, will I know what to do with myself? Will I know how to live again? I don't remember what it feels like to *not* be nauseous. I really don't. Will I know how to interact with people? Will I know how to go to the grocery store or drive down the street feeling safe, warm and happy? I just feel scared now. Scared of what hell life has to offer, what hell is lurking in the shadows. Illness-related post traumatic stress disorder, here I come.

Tuesday, February 24, 2004

I am sick. I caught the puke flu—again. I am so sick of being sick. Puking and can't eat. Gee, I haven't had enough of that.

I am kind of despairing.

Elise seems to be OK. Thanks for your prayers.

Wednesday, February 25, 2004

My fever broke last night for the first time in a couple of days. No puking so far today. Stomach rolling like the sea. I'm going to try to eat some apple sauce for lunch. I had some juice this morning for the first time in a while. Been drinking Gatorade. Yuck.

Had some anxiety last night. Here in the dark unable to go to sleep. I got restless. Tried to stifle the anxiety by turning on the TV. It was after 1 A.M. and Twilight Zone was on. It was the one with the piano that played music that would expose the true feelings of the listener. It was "eh" as far as Twilight Zones go. I fell asleep at some point, thank God.

Tomorrow I go to see Dr. Keanu and also to a lab to get a diabetes test. You know, the one where you drink the orange soda? I remember really liking the stuff last time, but this time I think I will be too sick to like it and may even puke it up. But I will try not to do that whole Pygmalion thing and predispose myself to such a happening.

I don't mean to complain, but IS THIS PREGNANCY OVER YET?!?

Ugh.

Friday, February 27, 2004

I didn't puke day before yesterday but couldn't really eat. Yesterday I puked my head off and the runs just got runnier. Today I haven't puked yet but the runnier runs are worse than ever with a new pastel makeover just in time for spring.

I was only able to take in three cups of fluid yesterday, but so far I have had nearly four and a half today. If I can't get down all six I am going to triage for IVs. Every time I take a sip my stomach starts grumbling, and I have to run to the toilet. Lovely. I hope Elise is oblivious to all this. I'm sure she's hungry as I have absolutely no nutritional stores after all those months of severe HG. She's still beating me senseless, so I suppose all is well. This morning she nearly kicked me out of bed, but after waking up fully I realized she had the hiccups and must have had them for quite some time, because she was already thoroughly, violently annoyed. I can always tell, because she starts playing my guts like a harp.

Yesterday I went in for the gestational diabetes test. I drank the orange soda and kept it down! Went to see Dr. Keanu after that. He has a pockmark right in the middle of his forehead just like I do. We are twins separated at birth.

Because of the incompetent cervix my husband will usually enter the waiting room before me and ask one of the normal patients if they mind giving up their seat on the couch so that his sick wife with the incompetent cervix may come in to lie down and wait so as not to endanger the baby. No one has ever declined to offer their compassion or their place on the couch. Charitably, they move to the comfortable chairs. Today was the same. However, Dr. Keanu asked us if we would start coming on Fridays at a certain time when there were hardly any patients so that I could have clear access to the couch and more time for my appointments. He also mentioned that the reason he asked was because the nice, very healthy lady, who so graciously donated her seat, complained.

It's disappointing to learn that there are people in the world who care more about their big fat comfortable arse than they care about the safety of your child or comforting you when you are in misery and they are not. The woman saw me when I came in and got on the couch; I looked like *crap* from all this vomiting, diarrhea and bed rest. She looked rosy cheeked and happy and when I asked, my doctor's countenance confirmed that she was indeed a healthy patient. Then I got kind of annoyed at him for even mentioning it. Like I haven't been through enough! I thought that perhaps it might have been more reasonable (and compassionate) of him to simply say, "Hey, can you come on Fridays from now on? Friday is a good day for me, and you'll have more time and access to the couch." Instead I was told I was a pain in someone's rear and was asked to alter my life to make part of a healthy person's pregnancy more pleasant!

I said, "Look, we asked if she would donate her seat, she willingly did so, and now she is mad at us? If she didn't want to give up her seat for a sick person then she should have just said 'Heck no, you can't have my seat!'" I then told Dr. Keanu that he had done his business of asking but the answer was no; I would not change my schedule to accommodate other people who get mad about their own, feigned compassion. My husband abruptly interrupted my "furthermore" saying we would come on Fridays. Keanu looked relieved, and I gave up arguing at that point. It was not a hill I wanted to die on.

On the way out, two nurses and a receptionist were very rude to us. We ignored the nurses, but by the time we got to the receptionist my husband had had it. She wanted to know how much our co-pay was because she doesn't ever seem to know what she is supposed to charge patients. My husband told her we didn't have a co-pay at which point she started to argue with him that surely we had a co-pay, which we don't and we know we don't from talking with our insurance, something she obviously has not bothered to do. She wanted us to pay the co-pay and then work any refund out with our insurance. She has been doing this for a while and we have nearly a hundred dollars coming to us that, months later, we still don't have, so my husband said that he was not going to continue to pay and that she needed to do her job because he was sick of doing it for her. He told her that he was totally stressed out with a sick wife and a child to take care of and that he was not going to take care of her job too! On his behalf, she had been very nasty to him and has been this way since day one. He just had a Popeye moment where he'd had "all I can stands and can't stands no more!" It was kind of a rough day, and the second we got home I started puking my guts up.

I didn't really gain any measurement to speak of but I didn't lose any measurement, and I thought surely I did after all the up and down of vomiting and diarrhea. They're going to stop checking measurements at 32 weeks. Dr. Keanu measured my belly with a tape for the first time, and he said it was right on target.

I felt so bad yesterday I couldn't even get on the computer. You *know* I feel bad when I don't sign on for a good measure of public whining!

Last week I was boohooing about wanting to get out of bed. You'll be glad to know that I have been put back in my place and will be very happy just to be able to eat again. This pregnancy is a constant humbling. I can only imagine, daydream about the day, so far from now, when I will "belong to myself" again and be able to eat without any concern that I might not be able to hold it down. I do remember a day a long time ago when that was possible, when I ate without even thinking. Those were good days physically speaking!

That's about all I have to tell except for the neat thing that happened the other day. Elise was being rambunctious, and I heard her little bone pop through my tummy. You know, like when you get up and your leg pops? That's what she did. She was moving around, and I heard this little muffled pop. Very cute.

In a few days we will go and get our 4D sonogram. Perhaps I should reschedule it for Friday so as not to *bother* any healthy people with my suffering. Hello, can you say Leo DiCaprio's character in *The Beach*?! UGH!

March

Monday, March 01, 2004

I woke up at around 4 A.M. when Tee-tee Boy got up to use the potty. His daddy wakes him up to go so he won't go in the bed. Little One cries all the way to the potty and back. Heehee! Anyway, all the fussin' woke me up, and I couldn't go back to sleep.

Here in the darkness the mind starts working and takes me places sometimes that I do not want to go. I turned on the radio and got on the laptop and surfed until I *finally* found the Carter's side-snap baby undershirts I have been scouring the surface of the earth for.

Ugh, Butterfly Kisses is on the radio. Way too sappy.

I think part of the reason I can't sleep is because in three hours or so the plan is to see Elise's face for the first time. Today's the day for the 4D ultrasound. They're going to give me a disk of jpgs, so you too might see Elise today!

Wella, wella...It's still not quite six in the morning, so I guess maybe I'll try to catch one or two winks before the big event. I'm sort of dreading going to the office a little bit because everyone is so dang grumpy there all the time, and yes, I have every intention of asking a healthy person if I may have her seat on the couch.

My MIL is taking me because my husband has taken so much time off of work that he is starting to get nervous. It will be good for her to see Elise before she is born and doubly good for her to take some pictures back to my FIL, a preacher, who has told me such things as "Abortion isn't my issue," and "It's not a baby until it comes out crying." My husband says his dad doesn't really mean these things and that he's just protecting himself because he lost his grandchild in an abortion. My MIL once told my husband that ending the life of a gestating child is "a choice between a woman and 'her' god." That may be, but the one and only God has told us which choice is acceptable to Him.

"This day I call the heavens and the earth as witnesses against you that I have set before you life and death, blessings and curses. Now choose life, so that you and your children may live." Deut. 30:19

Dealing with my in-laws' perspectives has been deeply, personally painful for my husband and me, and in the context of preachers, Christianity and God, I have to say that I wish I could make this avid, church-going couple really care about these little people, created by God's own Hand.

"Did not he who made me in the womb make them? Did not the same one form us both within our mothers?" Job 31:15

By His own Word God calls children His reward.

"Children are a heritage from the LORD, offspring a reward from Him." Psalm 127:3

Further, I wish that everyone who professes faith in Christ could accept that our bodies do not belong to us.

"Do you not know that your bodies are temples of the Holy Spirit, who is in you, whom you have received from God? You are not your own; you were bought at a price. Therefore honor God with your bodies." 1 Corinthians 6:19-20

One who bears the mark of Christ upon her soul can only advocate the choice that God advocates—even when the temptation to escape a crisis pregnancy is *overwhelming*. When

God compels His children: *"Love your neighbor as yourself,"* (Mark 12:31), He advocates the choice of love.

"Love is patient, love is kind. It does not envy, it does not boast, it is not proud. It does not dishonor others, it is not self-seeking, it is not easily angered, it keeps no record of wrongs. Love does not delight in evil but rejoices with the truth. It always protects, always trusts, always hopes, always perseveres." I Corinthians 13:4-7

And Love, ladies and gentlemen, does not make a woman a grave.

"For he did not kill me in the womb, with my mother as my grave, her womb enlarged forever." Jeremiah 20:17

Ben Franklin had it right when he said, *"Experience keeps a dear school, yet fools will learn in no other."* I am that fool. I supported abortion staunchly and yet was somehow simultaneously "religious" for 25 years of my life. Nothing any "lifer" ever said affected me. Ironically, abortion itself made me understand that if my child was a child they all are. And when is it ever OK to kill children? Is there ever a reason that really justifies it? When we see heartbreaking pictures of starving, suffering children do we think "bomb them" or "feed them?" What is happening to us? The shock of realizing I'd been duped by rhetoric and, appallingly, my own egocentricity all my life, combined with the traumatic aftermath of abortion, finally made me take notice of how contradictory my ethics were. And I learned what God really has to say *on His terms. It doesn't take the problems away, but it does convince me that there have to be other solutions. God's solutions.*

And I'll tell you one thing: When Jesus said, *"Let the little children come to Me,"* (Matthew 19:14) I don't think He meant for us to pack them into jars and ship them to Him personally.

Ben Franklin had another wise saying: *"He that doth what he should not, shall feel what he would not."* And, from the perspective of a woman who aborted her child, I would not want *anyone* to feel what I feel.

Later today I will see the face of my unborn daughter, and I will see the truth.

The Truth

Went for the 4D ultrasound today. Elise is a snuggle butt and snuggles her face into the lining of the uterus so you can barely get a picture. Already she's playing hard to get! I did get one pretty good picture though.

She is so cute! (No bias here.) She looks a little like her brother already.

We will go and get another set in two weeks. They're doing it for free since we didn't really have tons of luck today. Don't tell 'em, but I would have paid $200 for this one picture of her and been happy!

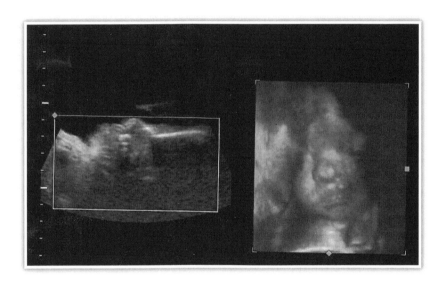

Elise at 28 weeks

The Best Medicine

Hey, folks! I am dying laughing! I don't know if they'll still be there when you log on, but as of right now, the two ads at the top of my Web page are for a fart deodorizer and morning sickness! Hello, but does someone know me?!

The morning sickness site just sells lemon drops and peppermints, so it's no big deal, but you *have* to go to the fart deodorizer site! I can't stop laughing! The absolute best part is the inset of the two adults *handling* the product! Holy smokes! This *cannot* be a real item. It cannot! Someone read it and tell me if it's a joke. I had to stop reading it because I was laughing so hard that I was scared Elise was going to shoot across the room.

If it's not a joke I'm going to buy a gross for my husband for Christmas! Though, after that last stomach virus I had it will definitely be a case of the pot calling the kettle smelly.

I am sorry, but I'm still laughing. Did you see the product? What's next? A pine tree on a string that you hang from Uranus?

Friday, March 05, 2004

Almost 29 weeks pregnant! Phew, this is hard work.

Same stuff, different day. Nothing really to report. Elise is kicking up her heels as I type.

"Hello, all you good people! Thanks for praying for me!"

Oh no. The windows are open and someone is burning leaves. Aargh! If I was normal I would like the smell. But I'm not normal. I'm all pregnant and barfy. And so I don't like the smell. And so—HELP!

OK, this entry is boring.

Here is some correspondence from this morning:

"Dear Husband,
First, WHERE IS MY MUSTARD? I CAN'T EAT SOFT PRETZELS WITHOUT MUSTARD! *I told you* this morning to GET THE MUSTARD! It's not in the cooler! Ugh!
Second, it's Fish Friday, so prepare to pick up some grouper Monterrey after work.
Third, you are getting spankings for not supplying me with mustard!
Love,
Ashli"

The reply:

"Dear Wife,
Uuuuuuuuuhhhhhhhhhhhhhhhhhhh!!!!!!!!!!!!!!!!
Heavens to Betsy!!! I forgot one thing this morning!
I'm lucky I have pants on.
Sorry about the mustard.

I love you, and have a good day.
:)
Hubby"

Hubby's Morning Routine

I thought I should clarify my husband's morning routine so you can feel even more sorry for him:

- get up

- bathe/brush teeth/groom

- wake smelly, bed-ridden cow-like wife

- take breakfast order and prepare breakfast before nausea lecture starts

- prepare wife's food/drink cooler for the day (remember mustard or receive harassing emails at work)

- dump wife's stinky pee bucket, clean, and refill with ice

- wake son

- administer vitamins to wife and child

- groom and dress crying child who is screaming that he hates school and wants to stay home

- prepare child's snack for school

- open wife's windows (so she can call later in the day complaining about outside smells)

- remember to supply wife with phone

- turn off all artificial lights before leaving for work as they "bother" ever-nauseous, ever-complaining wife

- kiss wife

- force child to kiss wife

- drive child to school

- retreat to hard day at work for much needed rest before returning home to begin grueling, evening schedule

Don't feel sorry for him: *he forgot the mustard!*

Saturday, March 06, 2004

The night before last I had a dream that I delivered my baby in an early induction, and they immediately took her away from me due to prematurity. Only, they didn't ever bring her back and she seemingly went AWOL in the hospital. They told me she died, but later I found out that they gave her to another woman who had long since gone.

Last night I dreamed I was an elementary school teacher again having a party for my class at my old house. Of course my parents were still alive in the dream.

We had balloons and were making "Bubble Buddies" like on Spongebob. We were eating suckers and having a fun time. One child, a boy, was emotionally challenged and was making holes in the ceiling by throwing his sucker up against it; the stick would embed itself into the soft ceiling tiles. I got angry and scolded him, promising to take him home and have a chat with his mother. He withdrew into a stubborn shell of silence.

I drove him home only to find that he lived in a wall-less shanty with no electricity or running water. Just outside the shanty was a smaller bivouac. Horrified, I peeked in to see a toddler sleeping on a table, only—was he sleeping?

I looked at his cherubic face and it was wrinkled, like an apple head doll, from dehydration. I was screaming that he was dead when he flinched. He "woke up" and told me his mommy was dead. I peeled away the flap that was the entrance to the shanty, and there she lay with the purple-blue mottle of death all over her silent face. Her legs intersected another pair of dead legs belonging to an older man.

The mother corpse sat up, and I begged her to take the little one in for fluids as he would soon surely die. She consented and whisked him away leaving her older son standing quietly at my side.

Needless to say, my concern over my mother's damaged ceiling tiles waned significantly, and I woke up with a heavy heart.

Monday, March 08, 2004

This is the first day of week 30. On Sunday I will officially be out of the 20's, and *praise God,* because honey, those 20's took about 50 years to get through.

Let's talk about anti-embolism stockings and leg hair growth:

When you can't wax your legs or even shave them because a big whale tummy is in your way your hair starts to grow making comfort in anti-embolism stockings an impossible dream. I think my legs itched less when I had chicken pox (and in the pursuit of excellence I contracted it twice)! Each little leg hair stands on end and pokes its ugly head through gaps in the fiber of the hottest leggings imaginable. The hairs hang there and at each shift pull. Hundreds of nasty little hairs being tugged on—not enough to pull the buggars out, mind you, but just enough to cause the constant discomfort of itching.

It serves me right.

Currently, I am the owner of a Sphynx, a "naked" cat whom we refer to as the "baw-head dog." This cat is lucky not to have hair otherwise I would torment it as I have every other furry feline in my history. Here's the job:

You take a furry cat who is napping peacefully and you find one single hair to torment. You grasp this one hair lightly and give it a quick tug, not hard enough to remove it, but hard enough to create the sensation of a solitary biting flee. Kitty bolts upright and scratches the phantom flea before settling into a blissful nap once again. At which point, you pull the same hair. You repeat this procedure until said cat goes into convulsions or you simply can't stand your own malevolence anymore. It's great fun, unless you're on the receiving end, which is where I find myself now. Cosmic justice.

The little gut monkey seems to be doing well, and by that I mean she is currently still alive and twanging away at my viscera. Praise God again! If born now, she has got great odds. She'd have to stay in the hospital for a little over a month or so, but she probably wouldn't die. This is good news! Each day she stays put elevates her odds.

Her big brother is growing ever concerned over two things in particular:

1. He realized on his own that his life will change—*again*.

2. He is pretty miffed that she will get nummy nummies, and he won't. They were once "his" nummy nummies and he's pretty territorial. He doesn't even particularly like it when Daddy kisses Mommy, so the nummy nummies thing with Elise is going to drive him bazoots.

I've got children's books to deal with concern number one, but so far I haven't found an Arthur or Berenstain Bears picture book on boobie envy.

I'm still looking.

Wednesday, March 10, 2004

The Fatkins Diet

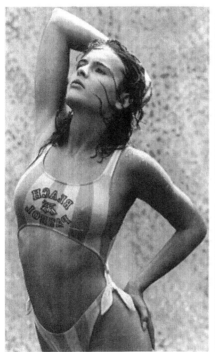
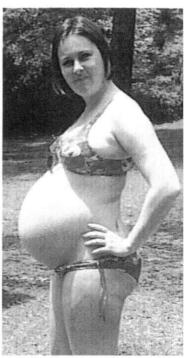

Me - Before   Me - After

*Adhere to a strict diet of Haagen-Dazs and Pepperidge Farm. No exercise. If you exercise do not expect to see results.

The days are crawling by. Ugh. I am so sick of being sick. I want to be able to eat something wonderfully pungent, my usual unsick fare, with confidence, without a care or even one thought of "this is not going to go/stay down." I want to eat with gusto! Lots of former hyperemetics eat like cows when they are well and end up gaining lots of weight. I can see myself being one of them.

I had always been 126 lbs until my son was born. I ballooned up to 197 in that pregnancy due to bed rest. After a year of no exercise and no diet change I found myself back down to around 132 or so. I stopped nursing when my baby was two years old (current WHO recommendations), and I shot back up to 145. I wasn't really happy with that, but every time I thought of dieting I would think of the three pregnancies and combined time of having no ability to eat and constant puking. Of course I couldn't bring myself to willingly forgo food then! So I accepted my weight and bought bigger clothes. I wonder what will happen this time. Wonder if I'll even be able to get back down to 145 without doing anything special. Dunno.

I started walking around our three-acre yard about five months before I got pregnant with Elise. That was fun. I think I dropped a couple of pounds, but I wasn't really trying. I did it to relieve stress and to regain some energy. I hope I can go back to walking, but I know I'm going to have my work cut out for me with two little ones!

Bed rest. How long has it been? Counting the time I *couldn't* get out of bed and counting the time I wasn't *allowed* to get out of bed, so far it has been around 25 weeks. *25 weeks!* How bad is it?

Yesterday I saw a commercial for the new Dow Scrubbing Bubbles toilet bowl brush with disposable head, and I almost cried because I longed to be able to get up and clean the toilets like a normal person. I prayed, "Oh dear God in Heaven, if I could only scrub the toilets!"

"What are you going to do when this ordeal is over?"

Some will go to Disney World—I will clean the toilets with an ear-to-ear grin.

Luckily, I have a new distraction: a stocking kit for Elise. I'm making one of those felt Christmas stockings for her. I made one for her brother when I was stuck in the hospital for five weeks. It was a Bible scene. A single figure took me something like seven hours to embroider, sequin, stuff and appliqué. I'm a fiend for these kits, *a fiend!* Elise's stocking is also a Bible scene, and it is a hoot to put together. I spent around six or so hours on it yesterday and got part of one figure embroidered and part of another embroidered, sequined and appliquéd. It made the day go by faster, and I thank God for the distraction; I am desperate!

I have nearly six weeks of bed rest left, and I am under the impression that when I get up it is going to make me feel better: less gastrointestinal problems and more ability to eat. I could be totally wrong. I really want to get up though. I have a few fears about that. She's lying a little transverse, and my water broke at home with my son, so if that happens again I am a little concerned about cord prolapse. But I know I just need to let all that go, because worrying isn't going to magically prevent anything! It's just extra emotional discomfort. I know, I know: "Don't worry. Just pray and be thankful." I try.

I *so* want this pregnancy to be over. I want my mouth to taste right again. I want to eat without a thought. I want to get up, cook, clean, tend my house. I want to be my son's mommy again. I want to go places and do things and be his teacher again. I want to go to church and make food to bring to prayer meetings again. I want to wash dishes in the church kitchen and wipe off tables and be a part of life. I want to go to cookouts and pool parties. I want to go to the beach and pick up a bushel of oysters on the way back. I want to steam them and share them with my crazy pals. I want to be a part of the organic coop again. I want to have play dates at the park with the kids. I want to function and encourage and be encouraged. I want to live again.

If Elise dies I will be sad for a long time. I don't know that I will even have the desire to do many of the things I now long to do—at least not for a while. But if she makes it, I will not be prepared for the joy. How could I possibly survive? How could I not swell and burst? I wouldn't know what to do with myself! Oh, to know that ecstasy!

(She is rolling around and kicking her head off as I type this. "Don't talk about me dying, Mommy!")

I did so much worrying with my pregnancy with my son. I had HG, the IC, the bed rest. They told me he possibly had Down syndrome and that I possibly had oligohydramnios (low amniotic fluid and relatively high risk of stillbirth). I worried my head off and when he was born I didn't know what to do because I had not planned for him to survive. Often I regretted worrying so much, but of course with my childbearing history and risks I understand why I did. Still, I have tried to give it up for this pregnancy. I haven't worried as much as I did with my son.

I try to be positive about serving the rest of my time. I try to remind myself that after she is born I will never ever feel the sensations of pregnancy again. And as I say that, I know that some readers will feel a blue pang because all they know of pregnancy are minor discomforts, wonderment and much joy. For me, I've never had anything but a horrific, torturous experience with a delightful little kick thrown in here and there.

I say to myself: "In a few weeks you will never again experience the "joys" of being pregnant."

I answer myself: "*Thank God.*"

I was in the tub last night and my husband, a guy who could formerly burn water, was baking his first loaf of banana nut bread. He came into the bathroom to ask me a question about it, and after I answered the question I told him that this pregnancy has taught him many practical skills. He replied, "Yes, it's true. But the biggest thing this pregnancy has taught me is *not* to get you pregnant!"

That about sums it up.

Thursday, March 11, 2004

For Elise

You wear me like a coat
A bubble in a bubble
A pool on a ship
Warm as Turkish baths
I move you
You move me
Synergy.

Friday, March 12, 2004

Pica rears its ugly head. Pica is Latin for "magpie," a bird that will eat almost anything. For me, pica started about a week ago. There was no suggestion or mention of pica. I just started having weird cravings and then remembered pica, which I've never understood until now. Pica is the craving of non-food items. I've never had this before and have to say that I *know* it's weird, but I simply can't help what I'm craving.

I would like nothing better than to sit down to a bowl filled to the rim with cat litter. And not the clumping kind either, but the kind with the big, shale-type flecks. Ohhhhh, nothing sounds better! I'd top it off with two new pieces of school chalk, white. I'd like to break a clay pot and nibble on the shards for a snack. I'd absolutely drool over a cup or so of those little plaster dooley balls all over the ceiling. Oh man, that sounds almost as good as cat litter! In between meals I'd just like to suck rocks. Mmmmm!

I know I can't eat these items so I don't, but if I could, believe me, I would! Instead I eat a soft pretzel with big pretzel salt grains on top and I pretend the salt is cat litter, yummy, delicious cat litter! I can't have much of this obviously, being that it's salt. However, for the moment it's delightful.

I go to the doctor's today, and I will ask him to test my blood for iron deficiency or some mineral deficiency that may be causing the cravings.

Pica is weird and just one more part of the extreme bizarreness of this pregnancy. I can't wait until it's over. In the mean time, what I wouldn't give for a heaping bowl of Tidy Cat!

Monday, March 15, 2004

Went to see Doc on Friday. Nothing much to tell. He said a test two weeks ago showed I am still anemic, but he wasn't surprised as I have had nutritional deficiencies ever since the HG. He tried to give me some iron pills in a blister pack, but I didn't want to bring them home as iron is one of the leading causes of fatal poisoning in children under six. He looked at me in cock-eyed surprise. "Really?" the father of a two-year-old asked. Oy! "Hello, how can you be a doctor and not know that?!" I questioned.

"Well," says he, "just put them where he can't get them."

"I'm on bed rest," I remind him, "If they're out of his reach, they're out of my reach, so what's the point?"

He thinks I'm just being difficult, but that's OK. He knows me by now. For instance, as I was waddling down the hall to the exam room I met him in the hallway. He looked at me and started laughing.

"Eh, what's the problem here?" I demanded pseudo-snippily.

He just laughed more. It's great to actually *like* my doctor!

Went today to try to get better 4D pictures. Snuggle Butt was snuggling even more than before. We got *nothin'*. I don't care. I think it's cute that already she's being "difficult." She is saying, "Hey, be patient. Wait on me. This is my private time growing with God; it's nunya business!"

The sonographer was truly sorry. She kept apologizing because we don't get our money back or anything. I was tickled. She said

I was the only one this had ever happened to and that all her other patients did very well on their second try. I'm so special!

Or rather, Elise is so special!

Having "stitches" in my tummy today. Uncomfortable. Hope it's nothing. Feels like something is ripping.

Hanging in there.

I have had an earworm for the last three days. An earworm is a song that gets in your head and refuses to leave. When you feel one coming on you are supposed to punch yourself in the throat to kill it, but I neglected to do so. Therefore, Who Am I by Casting Crowns is all up in my head feasting on my brain. Evidently there's more up there than I thought. I mean, *three days!*

Shoooooooot!

Tuesday, March 16, 2004

This is going to be short, but here are the important points of the day:

1. The gut monkey is still dancing.

2. My preschooler has informed me that he wants to marry the waitress from Waffle House, because she wore purple eye shadow and glitter last week.

After enduring years of his unfettered preference for Barbie, it is good to know that he is inclined to marry someone of the opposite sex.

I am now convinced that he liked Barbie because she was pretty and not because he wanted to *be* Barbie.

Thursday, March 18, 2004

Stocking work is all I did yesterday therefore, yesterday was a relatively good day. Later in the evening I started to feel siiiiick, sick, sick. Hubby brought home some coconut-lemon grass-chicken soup to die for. It was probably the most delicious thing I have "et" since this whole HG mess began. He also bought me some pad Thai. It was OK, but nothing compared to the soup. Still, later in the evening I had to get out Old Trusty, my blue emesis basin, because I thought for sure I was going to hurl. It freaked me out a little because I thought, "Oh man, don't puke up the soup and ruin *it* forever too." Once you puke up something you never really feel quite the same about it, no matter how delicious it was prior to puking.

My Little-little has started taking more self-directed interest in his gestating sister. This morning he came in to snuggle and he peeled the covers back saying, "I want to say something to Elise." I was pleasantly surprised as he said, "Hellooooo, Elise. Helloooo in there! I love you! When are you going to come out?"

We talked about her a little and he said, "I want two." I asked him what he meant and he said he wanted two babies. Forgetting he was five for a moment, I said, "Well gee, OK, I'll just get sick again and go live at the hospital with tubes in me for another year."

"Goodie!" said he, "Then we'll have two babies!"

I clarified, "The next baby we're getting is from Korea, not from me. *There will be no more babies from me, I say!*" And then I tickled his neck while he dissolved into laughter that ended the subject.

Ohhh, I got me some snuggle time this A.M., people. I kissed his little elbows and his face and neck and ears. He was laughing and accidentally bit my nose. "Hey, if you're hungry you need to ask Daddy to make you some toast, but *you can't eat my nose for breakfast!*" Something about that really cracked him up, and he laughed and laughed like I was the funniest person in the world. To him, I was. Your children make you a hero every day.

Last night I dreamed I was driving a car past the Coliseum in Rome. Inside the amphitheatre was a multi-level scaffold with tons of people standing in a white-robed choir singing Agnus Dei. We drove away with fading strains riding the currents of wind flying in through open windows. I wanted to stay, but my biological father was driving. He took us to a church where they spoke and spoke saying nothing at all. Then I woke up.

30 days left to my hell. I am wondering if something else will develop and I will have to stay on bed rest. Ugh.

You do realize that this diary is coming to an end. In few "short" weeks it will be over. There will be that much less of me to read, and we'll all be relieved!

Sunday, March 21, 2004

My son is sick, so we'll see how long it takes me to contract whatever it is.

I got up before 4 A.M. this morning. Couldn't sleep for whatever reason.

I'm feeling a little emotional lately.

Finished Elise's stocking yesterday. It's cute, but now I'm frightened and slightly depressed that I have nothing else to work on. Time will go slower if I don't do something.

Last year we kept some of the Christmas boxes outside in the shed. The squirrels got in there and ate everything including my husband's stocking. He needs one, and I *do* have another kit, but it's Santa and who cares about Santa? I want to get rid of it and make him something else with a theme more appropriate for the season.

We don't do Santa. My in-laws think we're nuts. We just decided early on that we didn't want to start out fibbing to our kids. This type of honesty is important to us. People are like, "OMG!" It seems to many to border on abuse.

If a kid never experiences the whole "Santa" thing he doesn't miss it. Our tot has tons of fun on Christmas morning, and we get all the credit to boot! Ha! A perk, not a motivation.

Christmas isn't "Santa" over here. It's Christ's birthday, but He gives us all the presents including the biggest one: Himself.

So we don't do "Santa." Big deal. Our kid is learning to trust us and knows that Christmas is about Christ. If it were about "Santa" it would be called "Santamas."

Love to all.

Tuesday, March 23, 2004

Email I received regarding Santa:

"You guys are so right about the Santa thing. My Mom and Dad taught me not lie. I was punished for telling small fibs. But they told me a big lie for eight years about Santa. I was *so disappointed* about there being no Santa, but I grew up of course and got over it. So many people forget why we celebrate Christmas. What would everybody do if all the stores closed and everyone's credit cards were declined? Christmas would be doomed!

My family has a tradition that everyone brings a tree ornament and when we all sit at the table for dinner my grandmother reads Luke 2:1-20 (the birth of Jesus just to clarify) and every time she says the word "the" during the reading everyone passes his ornament to the right. When the story is over, we get to keep the ornament we are holding. Everyone has grown to enjoy it, and it gives us a chance to hear the true meaning."

We're all hanging in there. Hope you are too.

Wednesday, March 24, 2004

Doody. That's what I feel like. The bizarre cigarette smell is getting stronger and more bothersome. I feel sick all the time, but this nausea is enough of a low-grade that the pukes are somewhat controllable with food and such.

I'm working on week 32. A precious friend and fellow HGer lost her son at 32 weeks. I always think about that at 32 weeks. I know not to apply it to my situation, but I do think about it.

Ok, journaling is going to have to wait until tomorrow. Itty-bitty is enjoying Spring Break and just got a Siamese twin strawberry in his fruit bowl. He is begging me to sign off so he can call Daddy and tell him about the discovery of such a treasure.

Ripley would be proud.

Thursday, March 25, 2004

It's still Spring Break. Itty-bitty wants to play a game, and I have already spent too much time on the computer answering email, so no journaling today.

Tomorrow I will tell you about what happened last night with the orange. I'm not sure if I should be disturbed or comforted.

Friday, March 26, 2004

More Spring Break. Will tell you about the orange tomorrow... mebbe.

Monday, March 29, 2004

The Orange

A week or so ago I was attempting to eat dinner when my little boy picked up an orange and lobbed it at my chest somehow. I say "somehow" because I didn't really see it happen. My fork was mid-way to my nauseous mouth when I was hit.

In my defense, this orange was a good size and particularly solid. Also, I am overflowing with pregnancy hormones and pity for myself. In addition, my son sometimes does weird things that make me constantly wonder whether he's normal or not, which is just another way I try to gauge what kind of parent I actually am. And I'm not always sure of myself.

So when this unexpected orange thudded against my chest I was so shocked that all I could do was cry. Yes, I started bawling because my son threw an orange at me.

I looked at him wondering what in creation had just occurred. He only stared back at me in astonished silence. I couldn't get enough air for crying (and because the gut monkey has taken my lungs hostage with her big ol' 4-pound baby butt).

A few seconds of looking at one another passed when he jumped up and ran to the bathroom. I heard him retching into the toilet puking up all his dinner.

He was so upset that he hit me with the orange that he became physically ill.

I have never been a puker (outside of HG), and it must take some powerful emotion to elicit the vomiting response. I didn't know whether to be disturbed or flattered. And while I don't know exactly what to think, I am glad that he didn't just sit there looking at me with no reaction at all, because that would be psychotic. Sorta like me.

Sometimes that's the reaction I have when he is in pain; I just shut off and sit there looking at him. I link this response to the HG-related second trimester termination of my first pregnancy, because a) it involves not being present to the concept of my children in distress and b) abortion is where that response began.

I need to be more aware of that and work to eliminate it. I need to push through my self-preserving "necessary" numbness 100% of the time when my children are in pain. I need to make sure I model the appropriate response so that my children don't become emotionless, orange-lobbing menaces to society.

Anyway, it turns out he was winding up the orange like a pitcher when the bigger-than-his-hand orb simply slipped free and went zinging through the air. It was an accident; he honestly was as surprised as I.

So that's the deal with the orange.

I am 32 weeks and currently working on the first day of not only the rest of my life but also the 33rd week. These last three weeks of bed rest are not going to go by quickly. My prediction is based on the fact that yesterday was a month long and thoughts of being mired to the bed all day today cause beads of sweat to pop out on my upper lip.

My husband tells me I'm in the last stretch and not to worry about it. And then he grumbles over tending to the "pee pot" when he gets home from work, so he sort of lacks that jolly sincerity he tries to otherwise convey re: the nearness of the end of this entire hellacious ordeal.

19 more days of bed rest (not counting the rest of today, and let's not).

I missed my vitamin the night before last and suffered cat litter cravings more than usual yesterday. I have found that Mylanta Mint Flavored gas pills have the texture of what I imagine is cat litter when crunched *and* the added bonus of chalky goodness that lately I love so well.

Tomorrow I will tell you about the tree outside my window.

Wednesday, March 31, 2004

"YEEEEEEOUCH!!!"

This morning I woke up at 3 A.M. with *such* a pain in my left, lower abdomen. I could barely breathe. I tried to turn over to make it go away. No dice. I tried to get up to make it go away. No dice; it hurt so bad I couldn't get out of bed. Breathing, breathing, trying to breathe through it. Scary. I called my husband, but I'm in an adjustable, hospital-type bed, and he's snoring away in the next room. He didn't hear me.

Finally, I was able to get up and go to him. The pain was awful but only on the left side. It waxed and waned just like birthing contractions, the real ones. For a second there I thought we were going to have to go to triage. They seemed to be getting better when Elise got very active. So much so that it scared my husband.

"Does she always move around like this?" he asked.

I didn't want to say, because if something is wrong, I don't want to be the one who said, "Everything's fine." She did seem rather active to me. She was rolling around and got the hiccups. She seemed agitated, but perhaps she didn't like being woken up to yelling and being strangely squeezed on one side. I dunno.

At any rate, I'm lying here in the dark two hours later, much better, yet kind of uncomfortably crampy at times, wondering what happened, how Elise is and when this all will end.

Elise hiccupped over 200 times before falling asleep, but of course, since I typed that she has kicked me twice and rolled once to let me know that she is awake and I am wrong. Oh boy! I can see the teen years now.

I still want to tell you about the tree outside my window. Also, the other day my husband suggested that I compose a list of all the unfun things I've been through in this pregnancy. I'll share that too but not right now.

I need to detox from the daily global wave of bad news reported by various online news agencies. I need to go and breathe.

Saturday, April 03, 2004

We're OK. I just don't feel like posting lately. Two more weeks in bed. I don't know what to think about that. Time is at a standstill, and I'm grumpy.

Tuesday, April 06, 2004

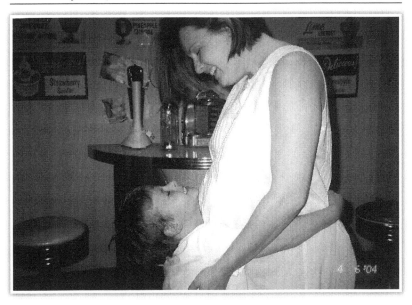

Up for just a second to snap a picture of Big Brudder in our dining room!

Thursday, April 08, 2004

The Tree Outside My Window

I've been stuck in bed for nearly 30 weeks. At the start of this I was too sick to get out, and when I was well enough to get out, my damaged cervix threatened my child's life, so I was not *allowed* to get out of bed.

I have a large window in my bedroom. Standing in front of the window is an adolescent dogwood tree. At the beginning of this pregnancy the leaves were changing from green to reds, golds and browns.

When you have very little left in life you cling to the things that graft you to the will to fight. I fixated on this tree. Like those flocked, color-changing weather predictors that were so novel in the '70s, this tree became my health gauge of sorts.

As I lay in this quilted prison I would roll my eyes towards the tree and repeatedly think to myself: "When all the leaves are gone I will be able to eat again." Daily I eyed the tree and daily another leaf would fall. The transformation to bony skeleton was slow for me and for the tree, but one day I looked out and there it was in all its leafless glory.

And I was eating.

Bed rest began with its myriad tiresome discomforts combined with the vestiges of an illness that does not want to fully release me until the last possible moment. I looked out the window daily and repeated the mantra: "When the tree flowers I will be getting out of bed." The tree has flowered, and I leave my prison in nine days.

Today I looked out the window and saw the "snow" falling. Wilted petals spread out on the ground like picnic blankets for the coming summer. The new leaves on the branches are tender and green. They are yet immature and possess still an unfulfilling sparseness. The days drag on and on.

When my window is green and my special tree dons her beehive coiffure I will be eating and drinking and walking and forgetting all that I have been through.

I will go to the tree, wearing my sleeping daughter on my chest, and I will tie a pink ribbon around the trunk for the world and us in it.

Tuesday, April 13, 2004

Here is a partial list of everything I have been through this pregnancy, ranging from the mundane to the not so mundane:

- four hospital admissions (two overnight and two that amounted to five weeks in the hospital)

- two trips to the E.R. lasting six hours a piece

- home IVs, blown veins, multitudes of sticks (including two occasions where it took seven sticks to place an IV or draw blood)

- IV bag changes, vitamin injections, tube changes, and pump managed by myself and husband

- four PICC lines (long central feeding lines that snake up the vein in the arm, through the vein in the shoulder and lie just outside the heart opening)

- two allergic reactions to PICC lines (involving phlebitis so bad I couldn't move my arm and complications with inserting the second line due to dehydration from the HMO's refusal to pay for the necessary mechanical pump)

- one bladder infection and one potentially fatal staph infection in my PICC

- one double lumen PICC insertion that became complicated and required several tries with trauma that increased risk of fatal blood clots

- embolism hose to reduce risk of thromboembolitic event (such as pulmonary embolism)

- blood draws most mornings for five weeks and weekly otherwise

- six X-rays

- a multitude of sonograms

- blood pricks to check glucose every four hours for over a month

- insulin injections, self-administered and otherwise

- bottomed out from low blood sugar due to too much insulin

- administration of >12 different drugs ranging from benign to systemic

- Zofran pump maintained for months (worn in leg causing painful lumps at sites, which needed to be changed by me every other day and involved self-sticking with needle/catheter combo to insert catheter)

- 11 weeks of no eating or drinking

- well over 100 vomiting episodes (I lost count) in 12 weeks

- vomiting blood, sometimes small, sometimes large amounts that caused clinical hematocrit fluctuations (involved one of my doctors wanting to administer morphine and put a scope down my throat and into my stomach to check for bleeding ulcerations caused by the wear and tear of so much vomiting)

- losing bowel/bladder control during projectile vomiting (and, due to inability to care for myself, having to sit in it for hours until someone came home to clean me up)

- liver dysfunction

- sludge in gallbladder (may necessitate gallbladder removal post-pregnancy)

- sluggish bowel/digestive system (due to inactivity from prolonged TPN feedings)

- couldn't brush teeth *at all* for two weeks solid, limited beyond that

- no real bath or shower for 12 weeks

- cervical shortening scare necessitating bed rest

- nearly 30 weeks of bed rest

- humiliation of potty by the bed and loss of autonomy

- ptyalism for months

- cigarette smells for months (no one smokes)

- bad taste in mouth for months (metal/chemical)

- scent intolerance for months

- vitamin k shots (during TPN)

- weird but horrible panic attacks caused by post traumatic stress disorder from prior HG history and current suffering

- Etc.

Thursday, April 15, 2004

It's Thursday. I'm telling you this in case you thought it was Friday. I know it's possible, because I thought Tuesday was Wednesday, and "Thursday" I was so pleased at how fast the week was going that I blurted it out to my husband who cruelly informed me that it was in fact Wednesday.

I could have died.

At any rate, here we are, *Thursday*, fo' real, and I've today, tomorrow and Saturday left. Three days to go. And if you don't count today, I only have two days left. And if you don't count Friday and Saturday, I'm already off bed rest!

Two more days...

I don't know how to feel. Approach-avoidance? I am numb. Two days. What does that mean? "Off bed rest." What? I don't get it.

I feel like Spongebob when Squidward tells him he has never tried a Crabby Patty.

"Those words...used that way...I don't understand!"

And I *really* don't understand what it means to *not* be nauseous. Somewhere in the back of my mind there is this suggestion that one day soon there may be a day where things don't stink, my mouth doesn't taste like industrial strength roach killer, and I actually experience no nausea. No nausea? "Those words... used that way...I don't understand."

Friday is Poodle-doo's last day of school. We're yanking him out because he's miserable, his teacher is miserable, we're miserable, and there's no point. Our home school will "officially" resume in a few months. Little-little has been talking about it and all the fun stuff we used to do:

"I like to do math things and get in the craft box and read stories and cook on Fridays and do science 'speriments.'"

My son, who hates school, *loves* to learn. His teacher doesn't believe this. He's a massive thorn in her side. He will not sit still, he will not shut up, he will not cooperate and participate in group activities because he's an extremely independent learner prone to self-isolation. He's sensationally social during play time, but wants nothing to do with it during learning time. Unacceptable, sayeth the teacher. He also thinks logically and has been encouraged to have a voice. And he's five, so he's a royal pain in the butt too. "Teach" has a military background. Oil and water. Friday is the last day of that. He has served his time; we all have.

Monday I'm taking him to a movie. A *movie*, I say! I don't know if I'll be able to sit that long, but by golly I'm going to try. We'll eat pizza and go to a movie! "Those words...used that way..."

Is this happening? Is this really happening? But I was just living in a toilet bowl, crying out to God with tubes in every appendage, pumps moaning and beeping, and an artesian well of vomit roaring out of my hyperemetic head day in and day out forever.

Part of me is still stuck there.

I'm going to need therapy maybe, because I still feel threatened by all of it. Maybe I'm a little angry. Maybe I'm a little scared, unnerved. Yes, perhaps therapy.

Elise is squirming. This morning she woke me up with her dancing. She was on a roll. It was a little unsettling so early in the morning, a little uncomfy. I thought to sing to her, and the moment I began she cocked her tiny unborn ear to listen.

Her body relaxed, her movements slowed to a stop. Her mommy sang lullabies. When I ran out of those I sang a song of six pence. She began tapping her feet. Too upbeat. I sang Humpty Dumpty and Jack and Jill: still good beats to dance to. I repeated the lullabies, and rest again she did, until Daddy entered singing his infernal, high-pitched good morning song. She heard him right away of course and started dancing again. She is a mess for Daddy. Daddy leaned over my belly and told her so and she kicked him right in the mouth.

"You're a mess!"

BOOP!

We had a good laugh.

Behind the laughter and the happiness, shrouded thoughts linger on the life and death of my first little one. Equally loved; I just didn't know how to get through it. Didn't know how to sacrifice myself entirely or how to demand excellent health care. It's something I can't resolve. A massive burden I have to live with. I don't know how but here I am breathing. Day by day. I take it day by day.

And today is *Thursday*.

Sunday, April 18, 2004

Getting ready for church because—

I'M OFF BED REST!

I'm a little frightened. I feel somehow that I'm losing control. I've been in bed for 30 weeks. It's all I know.

Been contracting a bit this morning.

I should be ecstatic.

But I don't know how to feel.

Most of this ordeal has taken a certain level of psychic numbing. Now I'm supposed to feel something?

Maybe my emotional functioning will be like my digestive system after TPN: sluggish for a couple of weeks before kicking back in.

I have to go now.

It's time to pick up my mat and walk.

Monday, April 19, 2004

Everyone said, "Don't overdo it," but I did anyway. I thought they were crazy even though I know better. I thought I could get up and walk around no problem, big deal. I thought that—not because it made sense, but simply because I wanted it to be true. It wasn't.

I went to church, went out to lunch, went to the grocery store, cleaned the toilets, made dinner, and thought I was going to die by the end of the night.

Church: Had to take pillows and "lounge" in the pew.

Lunch: Pretty normal but they put me in the seat farthest from the bathroom.

Grocery store: Had to use the store's electric scooter to get around and could barely get out of the seat, which I had to do twice because my husband was in another aisle. Bad pain in tailbone. Not used to sitting up. Husband collapsed in laughter at the sound of scooter backing up. "Beep, beep, beep!" That has been his personal joke all along regarding my big, fat, pregnant butt. To actually hear me beeping was too much for him to bear with any sort of public decorum. I laughed until I snorted like a pig in the produce section.

Toilets: Has been a goal of mine; "Oh, just to be able to clean the toilets!" Well, I did.

Dinner: For dinner I made stir-fry. My husband said it was too involved for a person in my condition. I poo-poo'd him and stood at the sink washing the bok choy, broccoli, carrots, snow peas, bean sprouts, green onions and mushrooms. By chopping time I had to sit down. During the stir-fry the back pain started to get unbearable. I plunked the tofu in, added chicken broth, corn starch and Bragg's liquid aminos and then limped back to my room without even serving. I fell into bed bawling because of the pain, and try as I might I could not get out of bed after that. Thank God for the bedside potty, because I couldn't even make the walk to the bathroom. I'm still feeling pretty awful today, which means no movie and pizza date with Little-little. I broke it to him last night, and he was so disappointed. A slice of banana cream pie helped. And I gave him one too.

On top of everything, I seem to have possibly picked up a bug or something while out. My throat hurts and I'm a little congested. Yae.

Church was great! It was about forgiveness, which is something I tend to have issues with. Our pastor told us a story about a priest or a monk or something. The fellow was counseling a woman who was having trouble with forgiveness. "I try to be forgiving, but I keep thinking back on the wrong that was done to me, and it still hurts and angers me," the woman expressed. The monk dude directed her attention to the church's bell tower. He told her that even after the ringer of the bell let go of the rope the bell still swayed back and forth ringing for a time. He said that possibly forgiveness could be like that; even when you let go of the rope and forgive, the bell of pain and anger may still ring for a time. I thought it was interesting and am still reflecting on it.

The biggest thing I struggle with is self-forgiveness. The pastor said we all know God forgives, but that doesn't make us automatically stop hurting over our regrets. He said the issue doesn't lie with God, who has perfect forgiveness and no issues, but with us and how we are able to receive the forgiveness. The pastor then told a story about a preacher who traveled somewhere on a mission trip or something. I guess I was fluffing my pillows and missed the details. Anyway, the preacher came in contact with some lady in a village who claimed to talk to Jesus every night in her dreams. Everyone in the village believed it was true. Of course he thought this was nonsense, and to expose her he said, "When you talk to Jesus tonight, ask Him to tell you about the sin I committed in my youth, the sin that haunts me to this day." She agreed and returned the next morning. "Did you ask Jesus what my sin was?" the preacher asked. The woman said that she had. "Well what did He say?" the preacher wanted to know. The woman answered, "He said He didn't remember."

And that's the way it is with Christ and perfect forgiveness.

The message was that some of us think we are so grubby that we can't step foot in a church or move an inch towards a real relationship with God. But that is the time when we need that relationship the most, and when God forgives He **forgives**.

"Come now, let us argue this out," says the LORD. "No matter how deep the stain of your sins, I can remove it. I can make you as clean as freshly fallen snow. Even if you are stained as red as crimson, I can make you as white as wool." Isaiah 1:18

Lastly the pastor said he hoped everyone would let go of "religion," a generic and fruitless concept, and embrace instead a living relationship with God.

So, church was great! I was a little embarrassed when the pastor acknowledged that I was there and that it was an answer to long months of prayer, but I was glad to be loved and to have such a caring family of people who have looked forward to me becoming part of our family life again.

I will never forget how they all came to my back yard and sang Christmas carols to me just after I got out of the hospital. I cried and cried and nearly disappeared on the spot, because I was so overwhelmed by their love. I went through such bad times but found a great deal of comfort in the Lord and in the people He has placed in my life because we all love Him and He is there for us and in us.

Church and lunch. Lunch was where my activities should have ended but didn't. I had a Portobello and Swiss burger with fries and pickle slices. I *hate* to be cliché, but the pickles were so good. I also had a delicious virgin lime daiquiri. My son told the hostess *and* our waitress excitedly, "Guess what! My mommy is pregnant!" I didn't know, but it seems he is excited and proud. His little feelings are so big and complex. Loving him is like unwrapping priceless presents that never stop coming.

After such a long day and pain that was bad enough to make me cry, I worried a little about Elise, who also was experiencing something new in my being up and doing. Yet this morning she let me know, by a few properly placed kicks and jabs, that all is well. She has drifted off to sleep and left me dreaming of her and what life will be like when she makes her debut.

The sun is lifting her head above covers; I embrace the breaking dawn.

Tuesday, April 20, 2004

I am sick and feeling like petrified yard dookie. Sore throat, dry burning eyes, tired, achy. Bed is where I want to be. Cruel irony.

Wednesday, April 21, 2004

I went to the Wednesday night prayer supper tonight. The pastor's wife, a dear, gentle lady and friend of mine, caught me sort of groaning over my aching back.

"I know how you feel," she said having just had a little one eight months ago.

Accidentally, I burst out laughing and said, "No you don't!"

She protested sweetly, "Ashli, I just had a baby myself; I remember the horrible back aches of the third trimester! I totally know how you feel."

"Oh," I said, "you were in bed for 30 weeks and then you just all of a sudden got up for the first time with a full-blown baby in your stomach?"

"Ummmm....OK, I don't know how you feel."

I'm a pain in the butt. It's a wonder I have any friends at all. That I do is proof of God's grace!

Friday, April 23, 2004

I am contracting lots this morning. Part of me would like to make it to May and part of me would like to serve Elise a gentle, loving eviction notice right now!

On a note of pure ecstasy, I must inform you all that peppermint flavored Tums, yummy edible Tums, are made of gritty, chalky, delightful calcium and talc!!! **Talc, I say!** I can eat four a day and pretend they are cat litter or chalk or any other culinary delicacy.

Going to a baby shower in a few hours. Presents! But more importantly: *cake*!

Went out to the shed yesterday to get the stored bassinet and car seat ready. The bassinet was fine, but the confounded, dad-burned, dog-gone squirrels ate through the belt of the car seat, so there's an extra hundred bucks we hadn't factored in to the budget. Well, that's it. I'm just going to have to send Elise back! Haha!

So while I was inspecting the car seat I leaned over and one of the pine trees dropped a cone or a twig or something on my back, ker-plunk!

"D'oh!"

I was too involved with the car seat to really be interested. When I put the car seat in the trash I noticed something wet and yucky on my hand. Must have accidentally squished a bug upon grabbing the seat. Washed my hands. Saw a spot of bug juice on my expensive, white, embroidered, big-butted, maternity nightgown. Great. Hope it comes out. Tiny spot of gross bug juice. Yuck.

Approximately nine hours later my husband came home and asked me what the heck was on my back. What? I dunno.

I took the gown off and came face to face with a giant splatter of set-in bird dookie. White urea and purple berry poop! It'll never come out.

I had to laugh, because I am a bird toilet. They aim for me. You have no idea how often birds have pooped on me in my lifetime. It's uncanny.

I think I was a statue in a former life.

Tuesday, April 27, 2004

Went to Dr. Keanu last Friday (going once a week now), and he said he was not opposed to inducing before the 16th of May, when he is scheduled to go out of town for a few days. Isn't this typical. I stay in bed for half my life praying fervently that I can hold in her little body just one more day, and then she ends up getting induced!

I haven't agreed to anything.

I feel a little creepy about induction. For me, it smacks of abortion. It is the same now as it was in my first pregnancy: I love her, but I feel I can't take it anymore and want her out of my body *now*. I don't like that feeling. I have it, but I don't like it and I don't have to act on it.

If I were overdue, that would be one thing; an induction would be for her. As it is, the idea is purely for me in order to regain physical comfort and to ensure that Dr. Keanu will be the one to attend. My reasons don't justify Cytotec patches and Pitocin. But then the day wears on and by night I am sometimes tearing with pain. Perhaps what I need at this point isn't induction but prayer.

I am having trouble sleeping. Normal for pregnant fatties at this stage of the game. I keep waking up at 4 A.M. unable to get back to sleep. Two days ago I asked my husband to pray for me each night, and each night that he has I have slept very well in spite of getting up umpteen times a night to pee. So pray, if you will, that:

- Things will be more physically comfortable or that I will have a greater will to endure it.

- I will sleep better.

- Elise will come on her own—but SOON!

- We four will continue to be healthy and safe.

I really do appreciate your prayers.

Nothing really super interesting is happening lately. It just feels like a waiting game at this point. I am still up too much, overdoing and paying the price. I need to work on that, I know.

Dr. Keanu gives me updates from time to time, telling me of the new cases of HG patients in the hospital. "She's not as bad as you," he tends to follow it with. "You're as bad as I've seen it." I win. I want my golden emesis basin.

My baby shower was great! Lots of loot and lots of fun. My teeth: the dental work that must be done after this pregnancy—I don't even want to think about it. I took a bite of the cake at the shower and nearly died. The pain was searing.

I had to have dental work after my son was born due to all the stomach acid washes from the constant vomiting and inability to brush. My teeth are worse this time around, but that only makes sense, because the pregnancy was so much worse. But teeth? What are teeth compared to nurturing a child and surviving, persisting, when I could have taken the "easy" way out. Teeth are trivial.

OK, lessee: Dr. Keanu, shower, teeth. I think I've hit all the recent highlights, which explains why I haven't been writing much lately!

Oh, my neighbor, who is in her mid '70s, came over last night with a large butter tin full of neck bones and rice! She also added a nice portion of tomato gravy on the side *and* topped it all off with some pear salad—sand pears from her trees of course! It was seriously yummy. This is a typical southern dish. For those of you who don't know what neck bones are, it's beef. You cook the neck bones all day until the meat is just falling-off tender. No one makes it like my neighbor Mama Birdie. I had already made lasagna, but once those neck bones came through the door we just put the uncut lasagna in the fridge for the next day. I mean, we're talking *neck bones and rice with tomato gravy* here! Boy howdy, do I ever *love* my neighbor!

I would like to say a special thank you to my favorite New York attorney for the Aristocrat wool soakers for Elise's little poopie-butt. These things are quite expensive and the thoughtful gift is so helpful. Thanks!

Elise is running out of leg room, but she is doing her best to say good morning to you all. She has worried me with a couple of slow days, but she is a child; she will worry her mother for the rest of life.

That's the way it goes!

May

Saturday, May 01, 2004

Went to Dr. Keanu's yesterday. He was walking down the hall to our exam room when he was called away to an emergency C-section, so no exam. Well, OK, nurse practitioner, but that doesn't count; she couldn't answer specific questions that only Keanu could answer. I hope the C-section went well and all is OK with the other mom and baby.

On Monday I will be 37 weeks. My son was born at 38 weeks and three days. If Elise doesn't pop out by then, I'm going to start doing jumping jacks.

Cried an awful lot yesterday; very emotional over first baby. Can't resolve it. Someone so special is missing from our lives.

Sunday, May 02, 2004

OK, I barely slept at all last night. SOMEONE OUT THERE FORGOT TO PRAY!!! C'mon, get with it!

;-)

Monday, May 03, 2004

It's nearly 3 A.M. and I obviously can't sleep. I try but I just fade in and out feeling weird and sweating like a pig. My throat is all fleshy, the delicate inner tissues profuse with blood, fluids and Bear Claw ice cream. It is fat and I snore now. I am a light sleeper and each snore wakes me up. In addition I am an artesian pee well. It never ends. Pee, pee, pee. I puked my head off after getting out of the tub last night, which still feels like today since I haven't been able to sleep. When the sun comes up I have to care for a preschooler all day on no sleep. I can barely move much less take care of someone else without having slept.

I am frustrated. I stopped trying to sleep and got on the computer. I read a vicious comment, the kind that cuts deepest, the kind that involves your health, your children, the stuff that counts. People can suck. I know that. It's just harder to put on my big girl panties with no sleep and oodles of physical discomfort. Instead I feel dismayed, crushed, incensed, outraged, frustrated, defeated. A chink in the armor; things are getting to me.

Children are a joy; manufacturing them is a nightmare.

When will it end?

The dove flexes tiny, nailed toes in limited, internal movements that soon enough I will never feel again.

"Hang in there, Mama.

Hang in there."

Tuesday, May 04, 2004

Full moon tonight, and I am hearing rumors. Rumors of gravitational pull and babies born.

For today, let us pray to the Lord, wish on a star, and hope on the moon!

I am ready.

Wednesday, May 05, 2004

The moon is bunk.

Thursday, May 06, 2004

A big THANK YOU to a special reader who totally surprised me with a neat gift on my May 3rd birthday! Totally unexpected but very, very sweet and much appreciated!

I am blessed to have so many who care about me! It is humbling and beautiful.

THANKS!

I overdid yesterday. I paid for it last night when I couldn't walk without assistance. So lame. No pun intended.

I went out for pizza at lunch and saw a gal who had been one of my home health care nurses. She was my last one, and I only had her for a few days before I got my staph infection and had to go back into the hospital. She was really nice though, a Catholic who prayed for me. She also had a son who, when younger, lived on TPN for years, so she understood the madness of living with a pump that constantly moans and wheezes and screams out its alarms.

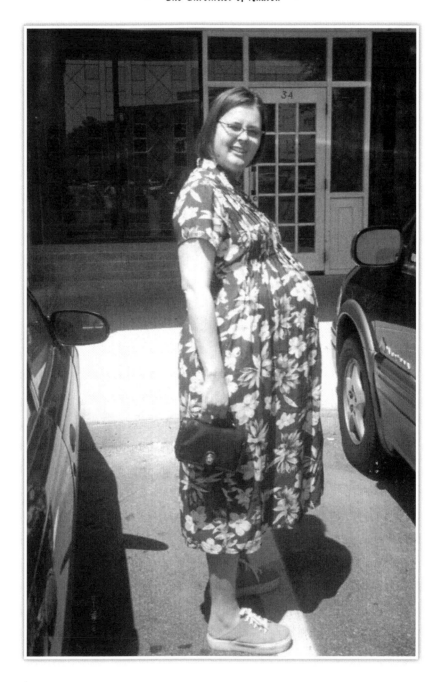

I remembered her name. I never remember anyone's name.

She was so glad to see me, and I was glad for her to see me too. It must suck only to get to see people when they're sick and never to get to see them come out on the other side. I wouldn't think you would get really satisfying results from your work as a home health nurse. The HMO gets rid of you before the patient is really all that well again, so I would imagine that most home health care nurses are out of the picture long before the person looks fit and alive again.

My ex-nurse seemed relieved to know that Elise was alive and well. Because of my former health status there was some question. I went through a lot.

A friend came over the other day, and we were talking about it. I started to tell her what nights had been like during the thick of it. It was just a description of living with various pumps and alarms, not the worst part of the illness, and yet, I couldn't get through it without bawling and feeling like the wind had been knocked out of me, without feeling like I wanted to run from my own words, my memories, the reality of what had been my life. I never want to go through this again.

Anyway, it was good to see the nurse so that she could witness the healing and understand that she had been a part of it. Maybe our unsettled crisis occupied a tiny little corner of her mind, and now she could sweep it clean with a happy resolution.

Elise is squirming around ready for her morning dose of Captain Crunch. We just got our first major organic warehouse delivery since the illness rendered that type of living impractical. My tot gets the Gorilla Munchies (organic version of Cap'n Crunch), and since there's still some junk cereal left I get the real deal. I relish any excuse to eat garbage, and "I'm eating four bowls of

Captain Crunch for the health of my son," is the best justification I can think of.

I console myself with the belief, realistic or not, that the placenta somehow filters out all the detrimental substances in breakfast foods and therefore I don't have to feel guilty for pumping it into Elise.

See how it works?

Tuesday, May 11, 2004

Guess what I got for Mother's Day!

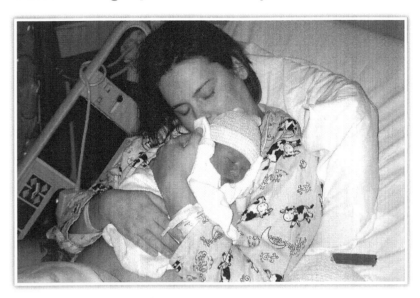

Let's go back a few days...

6:30 AM, Friday, May 7:

Another day. Ugh. Friday. Dr. Keanu would be going out of town at the end of the work day, and I would be anxious the entire weekend not wanting anyone but him to be a part of the delivery. With nothing to do about it my thoughts turned to Elise. Would I finally see the signs I had been looking for, the signs that reveal impending birth? With my son, I had a few days notice. The signs were there, and it was comforting to know the end of a long pregnancy was coming soon. With Elise, I didn't see any of the signs at all, and it was depressing, because I was ready—readier than ready.

When I woke up on Friday I was thinking about these things when I felt something. Nah, I didn't feel anything. Wishful thinking as usual.

GUSH!

Oh *that* was something! Aside from the full moon on the 4th, there had been nothing prior to my water breaking that gave me any sense that the end of suffering was near. But here it was! And unlike the trickle with my son, the Hoover Dam broke with Elise. I surfed the amniotic wave all the way down the hall alerting loudly to my husband and son that it was most definitely time. And I was freaking. I don't know that I really ever honestly anticipated that the day would come.

The gushing was such that I worried that Elise's head was not entirely blocking the cervix, which made me worry about cord prolapse, a rare but deadly condition. What does "rare" mean to me, the queen of rare illnesses? I know two people who have had cord accidents involving prolapse and it is heartbreaking. And it didn't help that I had stupidly watched a popular hospital drama on TV the night before that portrayed a main character's baby dying from a cord accident. So I worried. Which means I got back into bed and refused to get out. My husband threatened that he would call an ambulance if I didn't make my way to the van. Gushing. Terror. I stuck a towel between my legs and crawled to the van, somehow getting in without dropping the cord through.

We went to the emergency room where they put me on a gurney and wheeled me up to labor and delivery. Room six! There they checked me out and assured me that cord prolapse would not be an issue in my case. Feeling relieved, I got up and took a shower. When my water broke with my son I had contractions immediately. I wasn't contracting very regularly or very powerfully with Elise, so the shower actually felt great!

I had eaten a huge bag of organic spinach the previous two nights in a row, and let me convey that spinach, for those who aren't aware, is a natural laxative. 'Nuff said. Except that it was green. **Green**. Kermit the Frog would have been jealous. Dr. Keanu came in the door as I was coming out of the bathroom.

"You'll thank me in a few hours," I said.

"Oh please," said he, "when do I *not* get pooped on?"

I assured him, "Yes, but if you got pooped on with *this* poop you wouldn't eat all weekend."

My husband chimed in: "Corn poop would be worse than your nasty ol' spinach poop."

I disagreed: "No way. Corn poop is chunky and solid and you can get away from it. Spinach poop is slimy and green and there is no escape."

"And with that..." said Dr. Keanu as he excused himself from yet another of our family discussions.

Before Dr. Keanu left the room he tried to convince me to start Pitocin. I wanted to wait.

"OK," he reminded, "but I have to leave at the end of my shift 'cause we're going out of town."

I asked him how late he could stay.

"Oh, I'll stay. I'll stay and stay. *I will stay as long as it takes!* As long as it's over by 6 P.M."

D'oh!

"Oh *that's* lovely," says I.

"Well," he rebutted, "I'll stay as long as I can without risking divorce!"

I told him he had a choice:

"Look, you can get divorced or you can get *killed*. Take your pick."

He agreed that maybe he should at least *consider* staying.

I dilated to 6 cm without drugs. I asked for a birthing ball. This thing rocks. Literally. It's a big ball you sit on and it takes the pressure off your muscles and tailbone, etc. You can rock, bounce, whatever. It opens up the pelvic floor muscles and just relieves the pain of contractions very efficiently. I know, because they made me get in the bed once while I was contracting, and as we say in the South, I like to have died. "Get me back on the ball!"

After about 6 cm all bets were off. Drugs, gimmie drugs. I knew I could do it if I *had* to or wanted to, but I didn't have to, and I certainly didn't want to. I asked for an epidural and in the meantime some Stadol. Honeychile, that junk 'bout knocked me out. I didn't even get the full dose and down I went. Almost passed out on the nurse, but she got me to the bed before I zonked out. She was knuckle-rubbing my chest, the whole nine yards. My abnormal reaction shocked her a little. My husband explained how sensitive I can be to pharmaceutical intervention.

I don't remember much after that. About an hour or so is gone. If I got confabulatory, I don't even want to think about what I may have said.

At some point the anesthesiologist came in and placed the epidural. I remember not being numb and feeling the line going into my spinal space between the vertebrae. It felt very eerie and uncomfortably deep. I jumped. He gave me more numby and re-did it. Perfect—EXCEPT that it went *up* instead of down: my boobs were numb. My boobs were not having a baby.

The epidural didn't get into my lungs so I didn't have to be tubed, thank God. *But* the epidural didn't get to my cookie either. I felt everything.

Pregnant women will tell you that the urge to push out a baby is like taking the biggest poop of your life. They're lying. It doesn't feel like that at all. It feels like someone has stuffed a watermelon down your throat and is pushing it out through the other end whether you like it or not, whether you're ready or not. By the time it gets to the "outfield" it feels like it is ripping you in half, peeling you like an orange, and someone else is holding you down saying, "You can't breathe until you push this thing out, and you can't push it out unless you breathe!" At least, that's what it feels like to me.

I got cliché near the end of it, feeling that I just couldn't do it anymore. "Yes you can," doctor, student, and family lied. They told me over and over how near she was to being born, how close it was to being over.

"Two more contractions," Dr. Keanu said, as I pooped green spinach on him anyway.

"That's what you said *20* contractions ago!" I yelled in fury.

"Look," he said, "if you don't believe me reach down and feel her big ol' head."

I barked back, "I'm going to reach down and feel *your* big ol' head if you don't get her out of me **now**!"

A few more contractions, a few more pushes, a few more minutes of calling for my mommy, and out she came.

Then the fun began.

The baby nurses said something was wrong. They let me hold her for a moment but then rushed her to the NICU. She was "juicy." Fluid in the lungs. The cord had been wrapped around her neck and there had been some stress. She hadn't gone without oxygen, but perhaps she sucked up too much fluid and it was preventing her from getting enough now. I cried as they took her away.

Moments later they came back into the room and told me she would have to stay in the NICU over night. They said I couldn't nurse her because it would cause stress. They said they were going to put her on continuous positive airway pressure (CPAP). This is not great news. This is what preemies have to go through when their lungs are not mature and they can't breathe on their own. It can cause abdominal distention and even a pneumothorax (lung air leaked into the chest space). It's just not something you want. I think I remember someone even saying something about intubation. I was *freaking*, seriously crying.

Someone brought a hospital food tray like I was going to eat at that point. "Oh, my baby may be dying, but what I want is a tray of funky hospital peas." I was still crying when someone else came in and said, "And how will you being paying for this?" and asked for my husband's credit card. Wow. Unbelievable. I wish Hubby had said, "Hey, can you give me a minute to process this jacked-up reality before you lunge toward my pocket for cash?"

The NICU nurse came back in and sat on the bed.

"You need to grieve," she said. "You need to be angry for what you have lost."

WHAT?! I thought Elise had died. In hindsight, I suppose she was referring to the loss of the "normal" birth experience that ends with a healthy happy baby and no NICU, but at the time she gave no clear indication of what she meant, and I didn't immediately understand.

"Is she dead? What is happening?!?" I cried.

The nurse said, "No, she's not dead."

I wanted to know if she was *going* to die then.

"I don't think so, but these things can turn into pneumonia so fast."

There must have been a two-way mirror. Surely this was a practical joke.

"Watch me make this poor couple lose it," I imagined the nurse saying to her friends.

I wanted to know when we would know one way or the other how Elise was doing.

"We're just going to have to watch her," the nurse said.

She left the room. I bawled buckets. We called our pastor and asked him to pray. He called our church family and the chain of prayer was moving. My husband and I prayed alone in the delivery room. After about 30 minutes of praying the nurse entered the room with my baby saying, "All is well. You can take your baby now."

I didn't ask. I didn't want to know. "All is well." Just give her to me! They told me she didn't have to be in the NICU, she could stay with me in my room, go home with me in the regular 48-hour time period, and that her swift resolution had been "atypical." Atypical, ashmypical. Gimmie my baby! Thank you, God! **Thank You, God!** For whatever reason, our prayers were answered exactly as we had hoped they would be. God is gracious, merciful and good. It isn't always easy to see that, especially when things do not go the way we want them to, but this time "All is well."

I took my baby home on Mother's day. A gift, a treasure, life.

This is my HG diary. Through it you got a tiny taste of what it means to suffer the severe, prolonged, debilitating illness that is severe HG. This account is still insufficient for the simple fact that one cannot fully appreciate what one has not experienced.

The HG in this pregnancy was awful. No, it was worse than awful. It was unthinkable. You will remember a time back in September when I was "talking turkey."

Abortion

Shudder. Shiver. My lip starts to quiver.

If one or two things had been in place at just the wrong time I might have done it. There were a few days when, if my doctor at that time (not Dr. Keanu) still performed abortions, I'm almost certain I would have killed my daughter. I asked him if he would consider it for a case like me, but he wouldn't. He said he still believed in abortion but didn't feel "good" about doing it himself. I could have stolen away, aborted at the local abortion business, but I have a Choose Life tag, and I could just envision that bizarre, shameful image. Think, think, come up with a solution to **get me out of this.** I could take a taxi. Yes, a taxi…

But then again, I didn't get the D&C when I could have. No. I didn't *want* to do it. What's all this stuff I've been telling people for all these years if not the truth? And how could I be sorry for the first if I went and did it again? How could I ask to be taken seriously by God or anyone else if I had learned nothing? I had to find some way to tough it out.

A family member wanted me to know early on that I could "do what I needed to do" and everyone would understand. Permission to abort. Horrible, irresistible permission. This person was trying to be "supportive." So many people offer this kind of "support." But accepting defeat, particularly when the life of a child rides on the battle, is the antithesis of support. Anything that separates the child from life is not good for the child, and anything that separates the child from the mother is ultimately not good for the mother. My husband, who understands these things, very clearly reminded me that I neither had his permission nor God's. He reminded me that God gives much and requires much.

"Remain in Me, and I will remain in you." John 15:4

I didn't *want* to abort, but HG is 24-hour torture for months. The flesh was oh-so-weak, and I wanted *out* of the devastating illness, so I definitely thought about it. My pastor came and talked to me. You will remember that conversation from my diary entry in September. Friends who know me, one of them a staunch abortion supporter, barred me from even *thinking* of abortion.

And God—wow, I hardly have the words to describe how God stayed with me. God showed me a way out. It was the way *through*, and it would be **hell**, but He assured me, *promised* me that He would never leave me. And He never did. And neither did Elise. And all is well.

Know that all of the support has been so comforting to me and all the prayers have been *powerful*. None of them were ever in vain. All of them were appreciated, and all of them were heard by our gracious, loving Father who, for His purposes, saw fit to bring forth into this world a little, living girl. I thank God most of all for His generous provision, and I thank everyone who blessed me by supporting me through the fire.

May all be well with you.

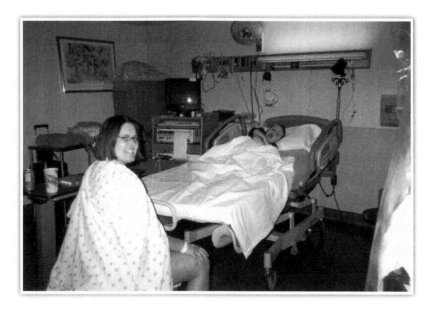

Sitting on the ball while my son watches Spongebob and pretends to have contractions.

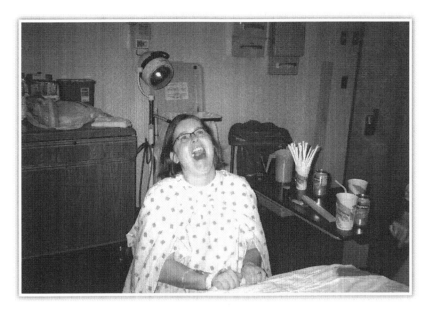

Yelling for drugs!

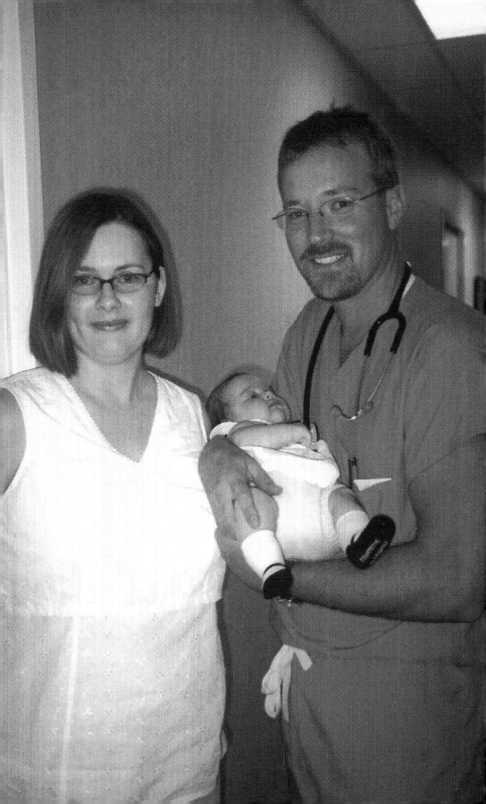

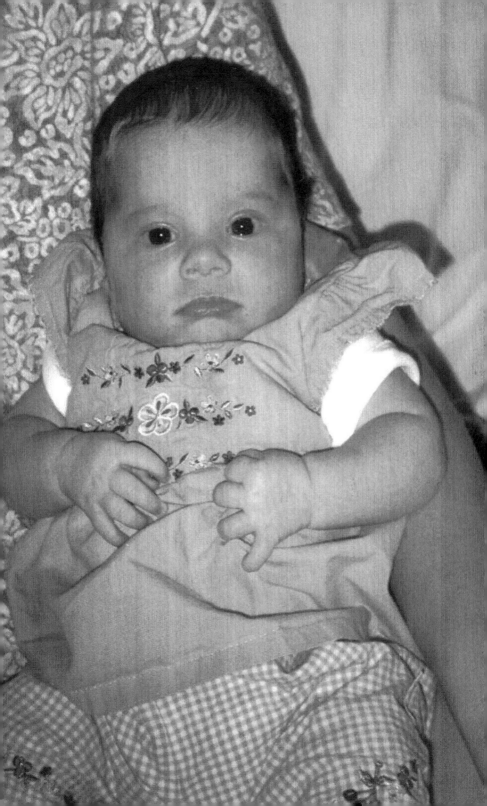

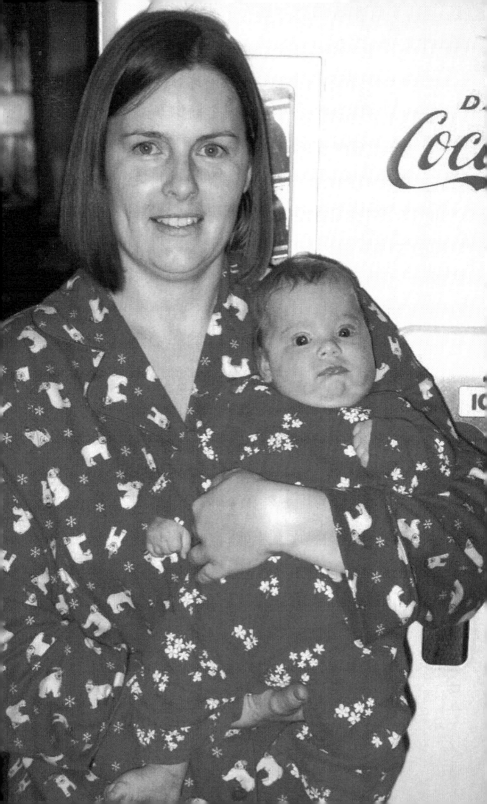

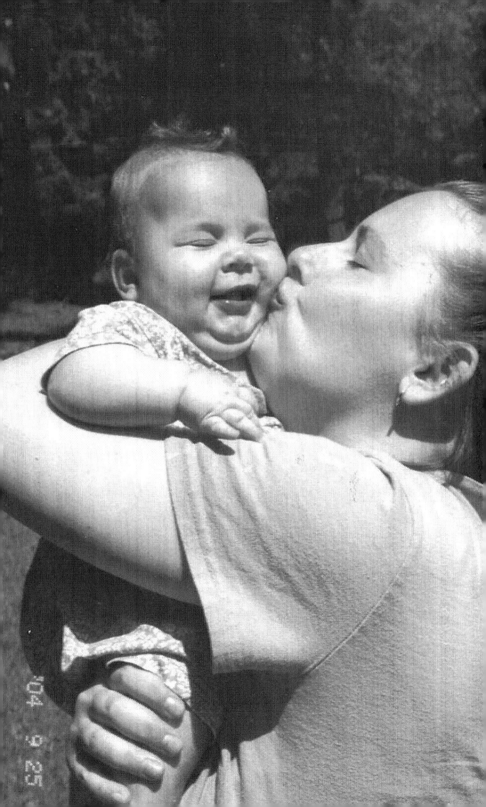

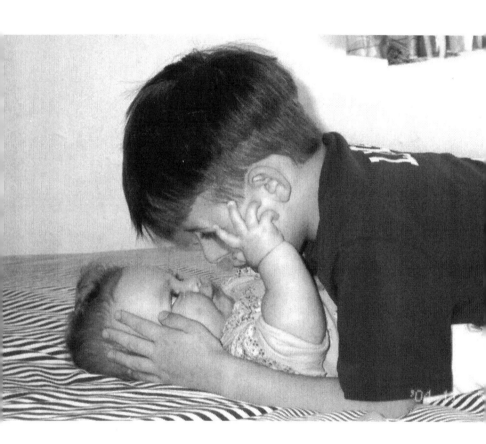

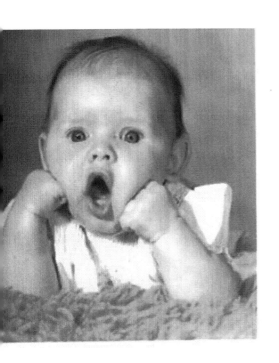

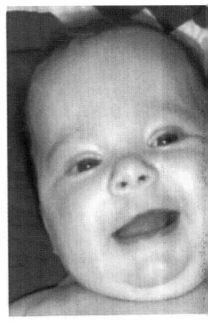

Mommy.

Elise.

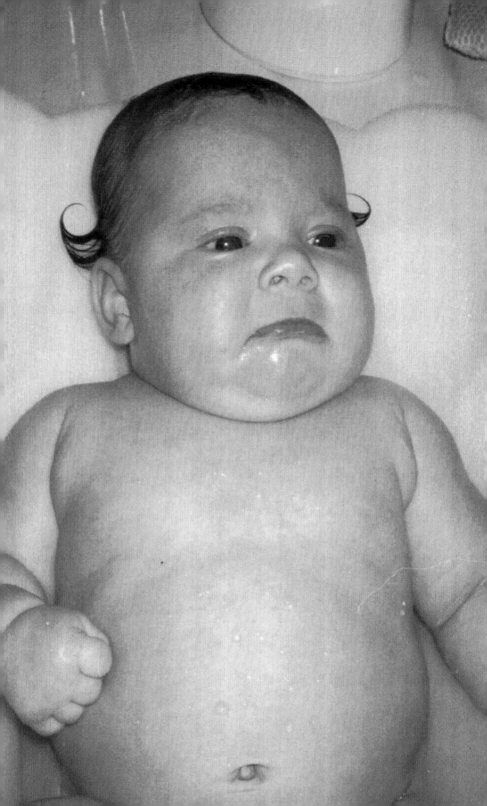

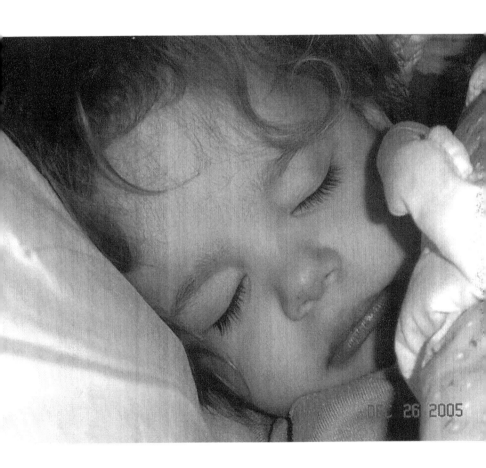

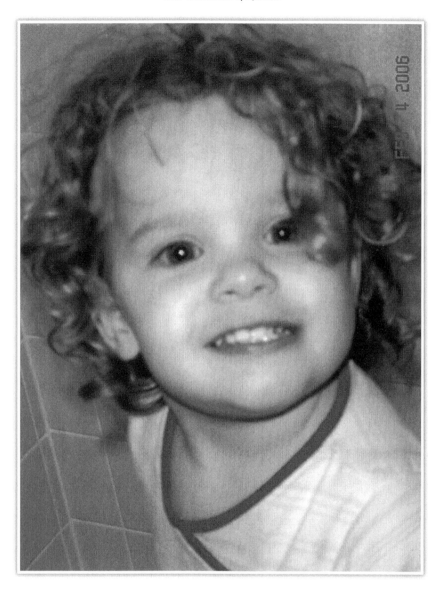

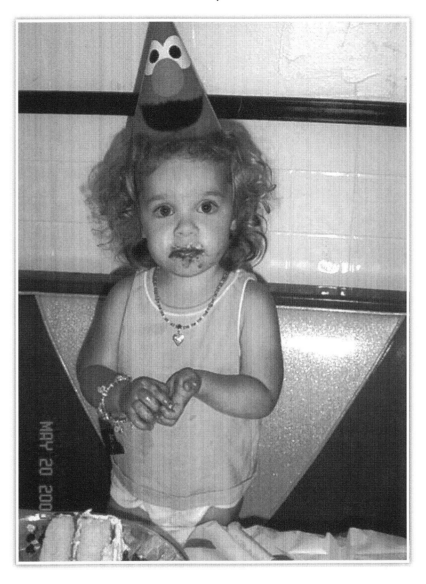

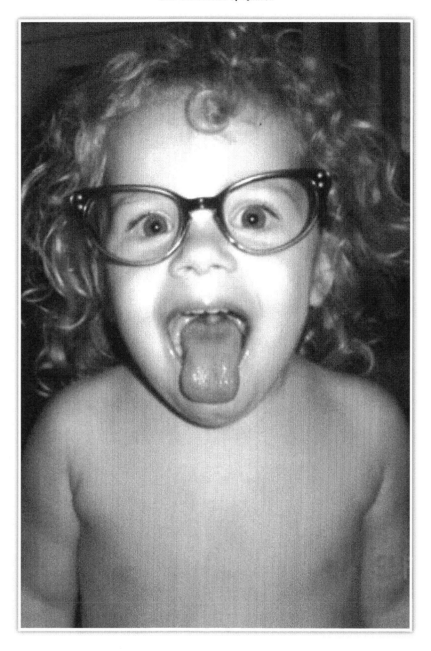

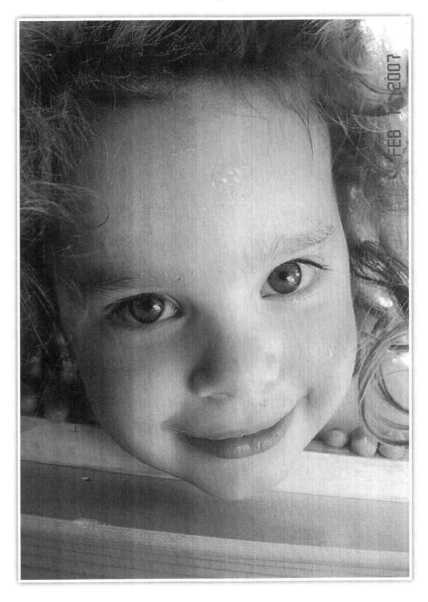

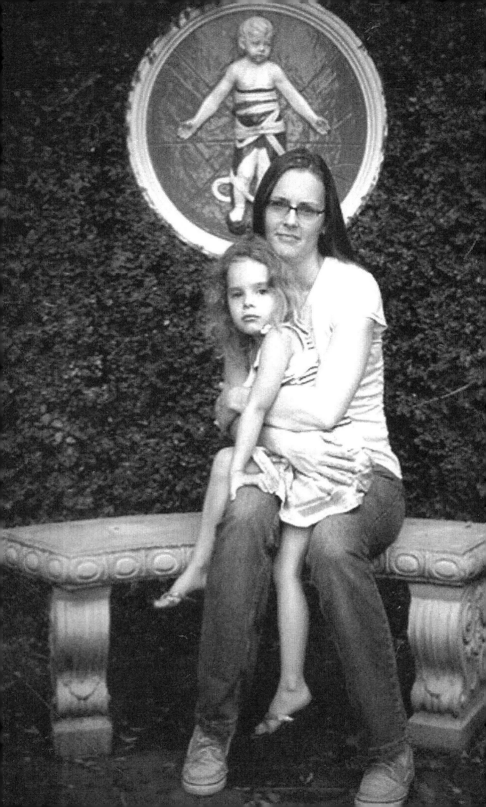

38926151R00128

Made in the USA
Lexington, KY
01 February 2015